HIV/AIDS and the Public Workplace

HIV/AIDS and the Public Workplace

Local Government Preparedness in the 1990s

James D. Slack

With a foreword by Chester A. Newland

The University of Alabama Press

Tuscaloosa and London

Portions of Chapter 2 originally appeared in Jack P. DeSario, Sue R.
Faerman, and James D. Slack, *Local Government Information and Training
Needs in the 21st Century,* reprinted with permission of Greenwood
Publishing Group, Inc., Westport, CT. © 1994.

∞

The paper on which this book is printed meets the minimum requirements of
American National standard for Information Science-Permanence of Paper
for Printed Library Materials, ANSI Z39.48-1984.

Library of Congress Cataloging-in-Publication Data

Slack, James D., 1952–
    HIV/AIDS and the public workplace : local government preparedness
in the 1990s / James D. Slack ; with a foreword by Chester A. Newland.
        p.   cm.
    Includes bibliographical references (p.   ) and index.
    ISBN 0-8173-0863-6 (alk. paper)
    1. AIDS (Disease)—United States.   2. Municipal officials and
employees—Health and hygiene—United States.   I. Title.
RA644.A25D564   1998
362.1′969792′00973—dc21   97-40918
                                                                      CIP

British Library Cataloguing-in-Publication Data available

To my beloved children
Sarah Ashley Slack
and
Samuel Douglas Drake Slack

Do not forget
the things your eyes have seen
or let them slip from your heart
as long as you live.
Teach them to your children
and to their children after them.
—Deuteronomy 4:9

Contents

Illustrations

Tables

Figure

Foreword

Learning from HIV/AIDS

Chester A. Newland

HIV/AIDS in the United States has been experienced most essentially as a personal and grassroots challenge—a mix of often isolated suffering and increasingly shared apprehension together with a search for understanding that has been both fraught with fear and constructively disciplined. Learning about the disease became the first imperative in the 1980s when HIV/AIDS emerged as an unknown specter, and learning remains the most necessary strategy for coping with it. The present book deals with one important aspect of this broad challenge: the grass roots of HIV/AIDS efforts among workforces in local governments. It probes the capacity of these governments to deal with workplace ramifications, providing in this second edition important longitudinal perspectives on learning at the front lines of practice.

The history of HIV/AIDS continues to have a peculiar impact on actions to combat the epidemic. Until 1981, this now globally dreaded affliction was a harsh but unnoticed intruder upon the most intimate of personal relationships. Then, for many long months, it remained nominally discovered but largely unacknowledged in the United States as a health threat beyond gay communities. There fast-growing terror and often unconcealed grief could not escape early notice and actions. Epidemiology and medical research quickly became linked via national networks, with initially hesitant but expanding governmental funding. Years passed before the surgeon general of the United States in 1987 mailed a message on HIV/AIDS to every household and before the National Commission on AIDS was created. But at key local levels, a myriad of volunteers, service organizations, and governments responded to deal with twin epidemics of fatal disease and fear.

San Francisco, the first government to take on the AIDS challenge, did so well before definitions could be formulated. The city facilitated networking by an array of existing and emerging community institutions and encouraged inventiveness in varied treatment and prevention efforts. Such twin necessities as compassion/ economy and prompt health services/pure research were quickly embraced, encouraged by grassroots organizations such as the San Francisco AIDS Foundation (SFAF). Local governments and states across the nation learned much from San

Francisco's experience, but leadership in New York City was also out front, as in the Gay Men's Health Crisis (GMHC), which devoted itself to providing health care to afflicted individuals and to developing social, economic, and political means to cope with what at first was a fearsome unknown. Learning and education soon became standbys of community action against HIV/AIDS in cities scattered around the country, *responding to grassroots realities of the time.*

Local governments in San Francisco, New York City, and other heavily impacted communities soon modeled actions to cope with AIDS in their own workforces. The national conference of the International Personnel Management Association (IPMA) convened in San Francisco and highlighted pioneering public sector programs. It attracted concerned local, state, and provincial government professionals from throughout the United States and Canada along with California health care professionals and concerned insurers.

Hope rose briefly in the late 1980s. Faith in medical science and pharmaceutical research was strong. The discipline of learning clearly worked for many gays. Numerous institutions embraced the challenges to learn and hoped to defeat HIV/AIDS. Efforts at the grass roots remained out front but with some philanthropic support and enhanced national funding, despite other public sector cutbacks.

But the grassroots battle against HIV/AIDS changed, and hope faltered. The epidemic quickly surfaced as a fast-developing heterosexual problem around the world, complicated in America by its spread among controlled-substance abusers. Learning models that had been pioneered within gay communities failed among drug addicts and heterosexuals lacking social connectedness. Agreement about causes of AIDS disappeared as complications surfaced.

Examining AIDS efforts both broadly and specifically, Linda Reynolds Broughton, former executive director of the Nevada AIDS Foundation, concluded that public administrators should heed the awesome complexities of HIV/AIDS and failures in dealing with them. She cautioned that, while "theories of learning in organizations and systems present learning as a guarantor of success," with respect to HIV/AIDS, it may not be one.[1]

This book demonstrates that local governments, while sometimes first in inventiveness and actions, face obstacles in their efforts to deal with HIV/AIDS in their workforces. The costs of health care, while pooled and thereby reduced in part through insurance, are compounded by burdensome sick leave and the requirement of accommodation. Many community residents and coworkers have difficulty, to put it mildly, learning to interact with AIDS-afflicted public employees. Elected officials and top managers also report their doubts and fears. Compliance with relevant employment laws, analyzed in this book, is difficult for many jurisdictions. Yet, hope endures, and positive actions extend beyond mere compliance.

Successes remain elusive, in short, but local governments have made some progress. True, we have no cure, nor has the cost of health service been greatly reduced. Inroads are also uncertain—and the prospect often seems dismal—with respect to the epidemic's spread among some American populations and worldwide. Hope remains strong, however, in terms of lengthened years of productive work and, in some locales, in terms of shared dignity in living and dying. Community grass roots nourish successes among public employees contending with HIV/ AIDS more than on most other frontiers of learning about the epidemic.

This book reports such modest successes, relying on surveys spaced five years apart. As its practical lessons demonstrate, local governments still have much to learn about HIV/AIDS. All illusions about easy or early ways out of this epidemic have clearly been shattered at the grass roots and by global realities. Nevertheless, some basis remains for hoping that, by coping with HIV/AIDS at the level of local government, we may promote and sustain human dignity.

Preface

RONALD BAYER wrote earlier this decade that the age of "AIDS exceptionalism" would soon pass from the landscape of American public policy.[1] To a great degree, Professor Bayer's prediction is coming true. HIV/AIDS, after all, is just one of a number of contagious diseases facing humankind in the 1990s. Many issues surrounding the retrovirus, moreover, have been "mainstreamed" into larger public policies and public debates.

But many aspects of HIV/AIDS make it unique and therefore worthy of focused analysis. The number of Americans with AIDS keeps growing at a phenomenal rate, even surpassing the number of those who died in America's greatest social catastrophe, the Civil War. The process of dying of AIDS also appears to be a uniquely tragic ordeal, primarily tapping the strength and resources of an age group that has much to offer society. The social and cultural stigma associated with HIV continues to undermine efforts to disseminate information that could end the epidemic.

Perhaps the most exceptional aspect of HIV/AIDS is its politics. It is the seamy side of politics on both the left and right sides of the spectrum. Who has killed more seropositive individuals by prolonging the epidemic? Democrats or Republicans? Liberals or conservatives? The answer remains unclear from where I sit.

The purpose of this book is not to "reghettoize" the HIV/AIDS epidemic as it was in the 1980s. The issue has become part and parcel of the fabric of American life and therefore should be viewed within the appropriate societal context. But I believe society can learn many lessons from the epidemic that can contribute to a greater understanding of how organizations and people might respond to other crises. With this hope in mind, I have in this book revisited the issue of organizational preparedness in managing the workplace ramifications of HIV/AIDS in the 1990s.

The present volume is the second edition of an earlier work published by the University of Alabama Press, titled *AIDS and the Public Work Force*. The new book has been retitled to reflect the substantial changes that have been made in each chapter. Chapter 1, "The Dynamics of HIV/AIDS," details much more thoroughly the particulars of the retrovirus as well as the psychology of employees who are dying of AIDS. Here students of policy and management will find information and guidance in dealing effectively with situations involving employees and job applicants who have HIV/AIDS.

I have tried to incorporate my thoughts on the workplace ramifications of HIV/AIDS in various chapters. Chapter 2, "HIV/AIDS, Public Policy, and the Public Service," explores more thoroughly the relationship among cultural considerations, the making of public policy, and HIV/AIDS. I originally published portions of Chapter 2 in "Responding to the Global Epidemic of AIDS: Cultural and Political Challenges Facing Governments," *Policy Studies Journal* 20:1 (1992): 124–134; and Jack P. DeSario, Sue R. Faerman, and James D. Slack, *Local Government Information and Training Needs in the Twenty-first Century* (Westport, CT: Quorum Books, 1994), 32–36.

Chapter 3, "HIV/AIDS and the Law," focuses on important nuances of the Americans with Disabilities Act and the Rehabilitation Act, especially in terms of their application to workplace situations involving employees and job applicants with HIV/AIDS. Some of my ideas in Chapter 3, as well as in Chapter 5, were published originally in "The Americans with Disabilities Act and the Workplace: Management's Responsibilities in AIDS-Related Situations," *Public Administration Review* 55:4 (July/August 1995): 365–370.

Chapter 4, "Attitudes toward HIV/AIDS in the Workplace," and Chapter 5, "Workplace Policies and Procedures," are both based on new survey data with a greater focus on the issue of reasonable accommodation for job applicants and employees with HIV/AIDS. I published portions of these chapters originally in "Workplace Preparedness and the Americans with Disabilities Act: Lessons from Municipal Government's Management of HIV/AIDS," *Public Administration Review* 56:2 (March/April 1996): 159–167.

The final chapter, "HIV/AIDS and the Public Service: The Crisis Revisited," takes a fresher and more detailed look at how organizations can become proactive in dealing with the workplace ramifications of HIV/AIDS. Portions of this chapter were originally published by the author and Anelia Luna in "AIDS-Related Documents from Ninety-six American Cities and Counties," *Public Administration Review* 52:3 (May/June 1992): 305–309; and by the author in "Employers Must Confront AIDS Issue," in *Crain's Cleveland Business* 13 (April 27, 1992): 11; "Mandatory Testing Would Protect Employee Rights," *Public Administration Times* 15 (March 1992): 9; "Addressing the Workplace Ramifications of AIDS," *Public Administration Times* 15 (January 1992): 11; and "Testing Employees for AIDS," in the *Journal of Commerce* 165 (December 11, 1991): 4. Some of the ideas in Chapter 6, and throughout the book, also first appeared in two government reports: James D. Slack and Anelia Luna, "A Model Plan for Managing the Workplace Ramifications of Acquired Immunodeficiency Syndrome (AIDS) for Municipalities in Cuyahoga County and Northwestern Ohio" (Center for Governmental Research and Public Service, Bowling Green State University, 1992); and James D. Slack, "Managing the Workplace Ramifications of Human Immunodeficiency Virus (HIV) and Acquired

Immunodeficiency Syndrome (AIDS) for Public Agencies and Health Care Facilities in the Southern San Joaquin Valley, California: A Model Plan" (Public Service Institute, California State University at Bakersfield, 1995). I am grateful to the publishers named above for granting permission to use portions of the earlier material in this book.

The data in this book were largely collected through survey research. During the summer of 1989, 526 city managers and mayors across the United States responded to a survey that formed the basis for the first edition. In 1993 the survey was modified to assess better the key issues of reasonable accommodation and undue hardship as well as to distinguish more effectively between *employees* and *job applicants* with HIV/AIDS when practitioners' attitudes and behavior were probed. During the winter months of 1993–1994, the modified questionnaire was sent to a randomly selected national sample of 971 city managers and mayors, of whom 520 responded. A copy of both survey instruments is located in Appendix A.

As with the first edition, I wish to acknowledge the contributions made to this project by several people and organizations. The following individuals assisted in pretesting the survey instrument: Dorothy Ball, executive director of the Southwest AIDS Committee (New Mexico and Texas); Tom Bates, city manager of Silver City, New Mexico; William Bowen, professor at Cleveland State University; Ernest D. Brown, coordinator of the HIV Project, Protection and Advocacy System of New Mexico; Jack P. DeSario, professor at Mount Union College; William F. Fulginiti, executive director of the New Mexico Municipal League; Robert Gallagher, city manager of Hobbs, New Mexico; Bill Jordon, executive director of the HIV Coordinating Council of New Mexico; Dana Miller, town manager of Mesilla, New Mexico; Sylvester Murray, professor at Cleveland State University and former city manager of San Diego, California; Ruben A. Smith, mayor of Las Cruces, New Mexico; Robert Stockwell, city manager of Alamogorda, New Mexico; and William S. Tilney, former mayor of El Paso, Texas.

Two student assistants were instrumental in collecting surveys, coding data, and developing the computer runs: Mary LaLone, who now is a public servant for the state of Colorado; and Kathleen D. Snyder, research assistant in the Applied Research Center at California State University, Bakersfield. Rhonda Castle, a student in the graduate program in Health Care Management at California State University, Bakersfield, provided much assistance in the research on legal issues and the scientific advances that have been made recently in the fight against AIDS.

I am also indebted to many people for peer reviews of all or portions of the book. Included here are several colleagues at universities across the country: C. Kaye Bragg, Department of Political Science, California State University, Bakersfield; Jack DeSario, Department of History and Political Science, Mount Union College; James A. Johnson, chair, Department of Health Administration and Policy, Medical University of South Carolina; Gregory Lewis, School of Public Affairs at American University; Everett Mann, associate director of the Applied Research

Center, California State University at Bakersfield; Sylvester Murray, director, Public Management Program at Cleveland State University; Norma M. Riccucci, Graduate School of Public Affairs, State University of New York at Albany; and Gerald J. Stine, Department of Natural Sciences at the University of North Florida.

A very special note of gratitude goes to Chester Newland of the University of Southern California. For more than ten years, Professor Newland has chosen to be my mentor. He has provided me with much needed advice, guidance, and support on this project, as well as on a number of career decisions. I am grateful to have known him and to have had the opportunity to learn from him. The field of public administration is, indeed, very fortunate to have Chester Newland as its senior statesman and advocate.

Several public health officials and medical researchers also reviewed portions of the text: Navin M. Amin, M.D., chair, Department of Family Practice, Kern Medical Center, Bakersfield, California; Hans Einstein, M.D., chief of staff at Memorial Hospital in Bakersfield, California; Stephen H. Hanson, center manager, Planned Parenthood of Central California; Patrick Hogan, an AIDS advocate and educator in San Jose, California; David K. Martin, AIDS Program Coordinator, Kern County (California) Department of Health; H. A. Pershadsingh, M.D., Ph.D., director of Medical Research at Kern Medical Center, Bakersfield, California; and Gail Sanabria, Title II Ryan White consortia liaison, California State Office of AIDS. I am especially grateful to David K. Martin and Martin D. Sharp, an AIDS educator in Bakersfield, California, for entertaining my many questions over the phone and without appointment.

In addition to Jack DeSario, two lawyers paid particular attention to Chapter 3: Roy F. Malahowski, Greater Bakersfield Legal Assistance, Inc.; and David Schulman, AIDS/HIV Discrimination Unit, Los Angeles City Attorney's Office.

Finally, several practitioners were kind enough to review parts or all of this book: Kathleen M. Irvine, assistant director, Administrative Service Bureau, Kern County (California) Department of Human Services; Kimberley Gallek, executive assistant to the director, Cuyahoga County (Ohio) Department of Children and Family Services; John Stinson, assistant city manager, Bakersfield, California; and Gilbert A. Watson, district manager, U.S. Social Security Administration, Bakersfield, California.

With so many experts reading the manuscript from a variety of vantage points, it is no wonder that suggestions and advice were occasionally contradictory. Considerable uncertainty continues to pervade all aspects of the HIV/AIDS epidemic. In instances where disagreement existed between readers, I sought additional opinions and eventually incorporated the suggestions that seemed most reasonable and congruent with other parts of the HIV/AIDS knowledge base. I alone bear full responsibility, however, for the accuracy and correctness of all information contained in this book.

The task of writing a manuscript is never a solitary effort. The professionals at the University of Alabama Press have always been good to me, and this time around was no exception. Ms. Marcia Brubeck, my freelance editor, was incredibly helpful; she chose to try to understand *my thoughts and ideas* as well as the words that I used in this book. I am especially grateful to the staff at the University of Alabama Press and to Marcia Brubeck for working on the book, and even updating some of the material, while I was convalescing from a heart attack.

My deepest gratitude goes to V. K. Unni, former dean of the School of Business and Public Administration at California State University, Bakersfield, for providing financial support and professional encouragement throughout this project. Members of the Department of Public Policy and Administration provided the intellectual and collegial environment that is always essential for sound scholarship: Jack Goldsmith, Thomas Martinez, B. J. Moore, and Phillip Paris. As always, the secretarial staff was incredibly helpful: Doreen Maddox, Diana Kirk, Liz Rojas, and Cora Starr. In addition, special thanks go to two members of the janitorial staff, Hernando Mondragon and Larry Morris, who made sure appropriate rooms were unlocked so that I could brew coffee when I arrived at my office at 4:00 A.M. to work on the book. Such consideration falls well beyond the call of duty.

Increasingly I find students to be central to any research effort. I want to thank my assistants, Erin Bauman and Rhonda Castle, for listening and responding to many of my ideas. For the same reason, I want to thank students in my class "AIDS and the Workplace": James Adams, Lorenzo Alverez, Martha Haslebacher, Theresa McClain, Rebecca Napier, and Elizabeth Rapp. Many concepts were refined with their assistance.

Finally, I thank my wife, Janis, for tolerating an academic in the family. Many weekends were much better suited to beach or zoo trips with our children, Sarah and Sammy, than to work on this project. Jan's love and support made those dreaded weekends go by more quickly.

1

The Dynamics of HIV/AIDS

THE HUMAN IMMUNODEFICIENCY VIRUS (HIV), the retrovirus* that causes acquired immunodeficiency syndrome (AIDS), has profoundly altered the way in which people view the world. Prior to the first reported AIDS case in the United States in 1981, people felt reasonably assured that American scientific capabilities could solve any problem facing society. While epidemics are nothing new, Americans were relatively confident that the medical and public health communities could control the spread of disease through effective strategies of prevention, treatment, and cure. We also trusted in the ability of government to protect both civil liberties and community health throughout the process of solving societal problems. Much has changed with the spread of HIV/AIDS.

With no medical cure or preventive vaccine on the horizon, faith in medical science has weakened. Confidence in the public health system has eroded; the number of people within the HIV spectrum has continued to grow despite more than a decade of aggressive HIV/AIDS education campaigns and prevention programs. For sound epidemiological reasons, and because of a wide array of misguided fears, people's faith in each other has also deteriorated. More than at any other point in our history, we are suspicious of the health of people around us, and we exercise far more caution in how we interact with them.[1] Because of the AIDS epidemic, the world in which we lived so confidently just a short time ago simply no longer exists.

Even our vocabulary has been modified to reflect concerns about HIV/AIDS. We are bombarded constantly with messages about the HIV retrovirus and associated diseases. We hear about the epidemic on television, via soap operas, and in public service announcements and commercials about condoms. Newspapers are filled with stories about famous people, such as boxer Tommy Morrison, basketball star Earvin "Magic" Johnson, and U.S. Olympic diver Greg Louganis, who have contracted HIV. The media extol other well-known individuals, such as tennis star Arthur Ashe and Pediatric AIDS Foundation advocate Elizabeth Glasser, who have died of AIDS. The disease is either the central theme or a latent element in a variety of motion pictures, such as *Philadelphia* (1993), *Forrest Gump* (1994), and

---

*Simply stated, a retrovirus is a microscopic infective agent that reverses the processes involved in building new cells in the body.

Boys on the Side (1995). The media have helped make the red ribbon, affixed typically to a person's lapel, the universally recognized symbol for the fight against HIV/AIDS.

As these examples suggest, many new words and concepts have entered into our thoughts and conversations, and they are often used interchangeably in conjunction with HIV/AIDS. People with the HIV retrovirus are described as being HIV challenged, HIV infected, HIV positive, or seropositive. Someone with HIV antibodies present in blood and other bodily fluids is said to have "seroconverted." People without symptoms are considered "asymptomatic," while those with "full-blown" AIDS are often denoted as "persons with AIDS" (PWAs) or "persons living with AIDS" (PLWAs). Someone with a CD_4 T-cell count of 200 or less, or someone experiencing at least one of numerous opportunistic infections or AIDS-related cancers, is considered to have full-blown AIDS.[2] Whether one is at the asymptomatic seropositive stage of the HIV retrovirus or actually has AIDS, infected persons are normally said to be within the "HIV spectrum."

Perhaps the greatest change in our lives is the realization that diseases can have political dimensions. Moreover, we have learned that the politics of a disease can sometimes outweigh the associated medical and epidemiological considerations. Such is the legacy of HIV/AIDS.

During its history AIDS has required local health officials to confront the politics of the retrovirus—HIV/AIDS–related bigotry and unfounded fears—within a multitude of groups.[3] In the 1980s, for instance, ultrapermissive members of the gay community fought to keep open bathhouses, centers of promiscuous and anonymous sex, ostensibly to protect the rights of individuals. At the same time, others chose to use the HIV/AIDS epidemic as an excuse to pursue legislation that would infringe upon the civil liberties of gay Americans.

The politics of HIV/AIDS persists in the 1990s and continues to take sexual orientation as its theme. For instance, respected newspapers in every gay community, such as the *Frontier* (Los Angeles) and the *Sentinel* (San Francisco), continue to exercise their First Amendment rights to print advertisements about local gay bathhouses and encourage personal advertisements from and for individuals seeking partners for casual and seemingly unprotected sexual encounters. Moreover, very few people in the gay community embrace the idea that abstinence should be advocated as the safest sex practice. Respected leaders in the influential gay rights lobby, representing well-educated and professional individuals with tremendous political and economic power in many communities, tend either to ignore apologetically or to defend unashamedly the self-destructive consequences of exercising too much freedom of individual choice in the age of AIDS.

Attitudes on the right side of the political spectrum also continue to affect the policy debate about HIV/AIDS in the 1990s. Homophobic activists demonstrate at Gay Pride parades with signs bearing such epithets as "AIDS Cures Fags" and "*G A Y = Got AIDS Yet?*" Key leaders in both political parties are quick to blame the cost and spread of HIV/AIDS on the immorality and irresponsibility of members of the gay community. Reflecting this view, North Carolina senator Jesse Helms has reinforced in his constituency the belief that the federal government should not allocate funds to fight an epidemic caused by "people deliberately engaging in unnatural acts."[4]

Local governments are also involved with the politics of AIDS. The decentralized nature of the American federal system encourages local politics to influence public policy on any issue. HIV/AIDS is no exception to this rule.

In Hollywood, Florida, for instance, some city leaders tried unsuccessfully to require mandatory HIV antibody blood screening for all prospective employees.[5] The ostensible purpose of mandatory screening was to limit future claims on the city's health benefit package and to reduce the amount of time and money that was invested in the training of employees who might then die from the HIV retrovirus. Also in Florida, Broward County officials were unsuccessful in their attempts to dismiss one of the county's budget analysts because he had contracted HIV/AIDS.[6] The fear of losing one's job, health benefits, and esteem among people in the HIV spectrum persists throughout the 1990s.

In some communities, however, concerted efforts are being made to quell the negative politics surrounding the disease and to develop effective and humane personnel and workplace policies. West Hollywood, California, was one of the first municipalities in the nation to develop and adopt a plan to protect the rights of afflicted employees. Many other communities have followed suit, some with the help of universities that have developed model plans to deal with the workplace ramifications of HIV/AIDS.[7] Furthermore, many municipal and county governments have created advisory boards to help develop effective HIV/AIDS public policies. These advisory bodies typically represent all spheres of local life, including people within the HIV spectrum, gay people, and members of churches. Local governments are increasingly searching for effective ways of controlling the political side of HIV/AIDS.

But the jury is still out. Today as in the 1980s, the fundamental question remains: "will reason rule or will the country be swept along in an hysteria that encourages policies in both the private and public sectors that are cruel and ineffective?"[8] Different policies, ironically representing comparable levels of cruelty and ineffectiveness, are offered by the Left and the Right. The politics of AIDS, therefore, hint at a greater debate regarding the basic nature of democracy—the rights and responsibilities of individuals and organizations—as America prepares to enter the twenty-first century.

Given the political complexity of the epidemic, this book seeks to assess the extent to which local government is prepared to manage the ramifications of HIV/AIDS within its own workplace. First, however, we need to review some facts about HIV/AIDS with a bearing on the American workforce. Specifically, we should understand the epidemiology of HIV/AIDS as well as the dynamics of death and dying. As the demographics of the epidemic indicate, this retrovirus can affect everyone: all regions of the United States, all communities within each region, and all groups within each community. The epidemic is particularly troublesome for individuals who are of working age.

WHAT IS HIV/AIDS AND HOW IS IT SPREAD?

HIV is a retrovirus, or a microscopic infective agent that reverses the body's cell-building processes and is thereby able to attack and destroy the body's immune system. Its action is called "reverse transcriptase."[9] Transcription is the process through which the body creates new cells while maintaining the same genetic code. "Normal" transcriptase entails the construction of messenger molecules made of ribonucleic acids (RNA) using molecules of deoxyribonucleic acids (DNA)—the source of the body's genetic code—as the template. The new RNA molecules carry the same genetic information to new and old DNA molecules.

The DNA-based molecules provide genetic information needed to reproduce the individual, to determine how the body should look and how it should function and respond. The genetic information transferred by RNA messenger molecules includes instructions for the production of a special kind of cell, the CD_4 T-cell. In large quantities (approximately 1,200 for healthy individuals), CD_4 T-cells are responsible for triggering the B cells needed to develop specific antibodies to fight off the invasion of specific viruses.[10]

A retrovirus reverses the process of transcriptase just described and, as a result, has the capacity to alter fundamentally the genetic message sent to new and old DNA molecules. In the case of HIV, for instance, viral DNA merges with host DNA. The body constructs messenger *DNA* (rather than RNA) molecules from *RNA* (rather than DNA) molecules that are already infected with HIV antigens, in particular the p^{24} antigen, which are the toxic parts of the retrovirus.

Using the infected RNA molecule as the template—as viral DNA merges with host DNA—an altered genetic code is transferred to messenger DNA molecules. The altered message instructs the body to accept the invading HIV p^{24} antigen in all cells and to let the antigen attack and destroy existing CD_4 T-cells. Hence the body's immune system is "tricked" into thinking (1) that the presence of the HIV p^{24} antigen is "normal" and "nonthreatening," (2) that an immune response to the invasion is therefore unnecessary, and (3) that immune responses to invasions by other viruses and infections are also inappropriate.

Upon becoming infected, HIV p^{24} proteins begin to envelop RNA molecules, and the process of reverse transcriptase commences. This is a gradual process, and especially when the person has a normal CD_4 T-cell count of 1,200 at the time of infection, the "new" message is not accepted readily. The incremental nature of the process helps explain why this retrovirus manifests in several distinct stages. It also helps to explain why it takes typically well over a decade for the body to accept the altered genetic message completely and fatally.

The Four Stages of HIV

The first stage of the HIV retrovirus is called "acute HIV." This stage occurs several weeks after infection when the amount of HIV p^{24} antigens in the body is sufficient to trigger an immune response by the CD_4 T-cells. At this point the body begins to develop specific antibodies to fight off HIV. Between 70 and 80 percent of infected people experience short-term mononucleosis-like symptoms.[11] The appearance of short-lived symptoms indicates that the DNA molecules infected with HIV p^{24} antigen and carrying the new message are still too few to defeat the immunal surge caused by the dominant CD_4 T-cells. In essence, the body wins the first battle against HIV. Within six to eighteen weeks after infection, the body even develops a sufficiently large pool of specific HIV antibodies to be detected by blood tests.

At this point, most people enter into a second, "asymptomatic stage" of the disease. While the retrovirus continues to multiply in lymphoid tissues, HIV-related symptoms are now nonextant. Infected people may become ill—catch the flu or develop cancer—just as noninfected people do. And like people who are not infected, individuals in the HIV spectrum who take care of their health will have relatively stronger immune systems and will therefore stay healthier in the asymptomatic stage.

The third stage is called persistent generalized lymphadenopathy (PGL), which manifests clinically with the palpable enlargement of lymph nodes at two or more sites that lasts for more than three months in each site. At this point, the balance shifts away from the CD_4 T-cells and in favor of the HIV p^{24} antigen. CD_4 T-cell counts begin to decline, and RNA molecules infected with p^{24} antigens begin to proliferate at an alarming rate. The body starts losing the battle against the HIV retrovirus.

The fourth and final stage, "AIDS," is defined in two ways. First, the Centers for Disease Control and Prevention (CDC) describe an individual as having AIDS when that person's CD_4 T-cell count falls to 200 or below (a normal count is typically around 1,200).[12] Second, a person is classified as having AIDS when he or she either begins to experience at least one of the opportunistic infections and diseases associated with this retrovirus or develops one or several AIDS-related cancers.[13] In this stage, the immune system can deteriorate to a point of nonexistence: a CD_4 T-cell count of zero and no HIV antibodies present. Death is imminent.

The Timetable of HIV/AIDS

The amount of time between stages varies, depending upon a number of factors: (1) the initial innate strength of the person's immune system, (2) the level of abuse or insult taken by the immune system, (3) the extent to which a person reinfects himself or herself by continuing exposure, (4) the extent to which a person has access to physicians who are knowledgeable about the HIV retrovirus, (5) the extent to which a person has access to experienced medical and health care facilities, (6) the effectiveness of the pharmaceutical strategy mapped out for each patient, and (7) the extent to which quality community-based services are available.[14] People within the HIV spectrum now often live more than a decade.[15] For reasons not yet fully determined, women seem especially likely to do so.[16] For a particular individual who had been infected in January 1998, acute HIV might occur in February 1998, with the asymptomatic stage lasting from 1998 to about 2006 or 2008. The PGL stage might then begin and last until 2008 or 2010. AIDS would most likely begin at that time, and the person might die between 2010 and 2012. A woman infected on January 1, 1998, might live until the year 2014 or 2015.

Taken alone, antiviral drugs can prolong life for only about sixteen months.[17] Several antiviral drugs that are taken in combination with one drug from a new class known as protease inhibitors, however, can produce a significant drop in the level of HIV in the blood system.[18] In fact these so-called cocktail therapies have contributed to the first decline in the number of deaths among people with AIDS and therefore give rise to much hope that they will greatly enhance both the life expectancy and the quality of life for many seropositive individuals.[19]

The realities surrounding the new drugs, however, keep the future uncertain. Access to protease inhibitors is limited in many states; in 1997 only 60 percent of Americans using other HIV treatments had the opportunity to try the new cocktail therapies.[20] The demand for protease inhibitors in Missouri was so great in 1996 that a lottery had to be used to select the seventy-five PLWAs out of almost three thousand who wanted them. Protease inhibitors also tend to be ineffective in treating approximately 20 percent of all cases. In addition, a strict regimen accompanies the use of protease inhibitors, and many seropositive individuals, especially those who are indigent and those who are emotionally unstable, have difficulty maintaining the course.[21] The slightest deviation from the proscribed routine results in the retrovirus mutating and replicating around the drug therapy. In other words, all drugs used in the therapy—antiviral drugs such as AZT and ddI as well as the specific protease inhibitor—will become collectively and individually ineffective in slowing the pace of the disease if the regimen is not strictly followed. Moreover, the resistant strain of HIV might then be passed along to other individuals who will find the same drugs to be equally ineffective in their fight against AIDS. These are the risks associated with protease inhibitors.

Modes of Transmission

HIV can be transmitted only through bodily fluids-to-blood contact with someone who is already infected. The primary bodily fluids that act as conduits for HIV are: blood, semen, and vaginal secretions. Since the early 1980s, only four activities have been found to be effective avenues for transmitting the HIV retrovirus: (1) engaging in unprotected anal, vaginal, or oral sex, (2) sharing intravenous (IV) drug needles and drug paraphernalia, (3) being born of, or receiving breast milk from, a mother who is within the HIV spectrum, and (4) being the recipient of a blood transfusion with infected blood or blood by-products.[22]

Fortunately HIV is incredibly fragile and therefore not transmitted easily. Even within the four modes of transmission, the situation must be optimum to permit infection. Oxygen and extreme temperatures tend to kill this retrovirus within a matter of seconds. Saliva also helps deter the HIV p^{24} antigen. There are no documented cases of infection through casual contact with someone who has HIV as there are with tuberculosis.

Open cuts, sores, and other causes of bleeding are essential for transmission of HIV.[23] This fact helps explain the different ways in which the retrovirus is contracted. HIV is more prevalent among heterosexuals in Africa, for instance, because an unchecked epidemic of venereal disease has produced an abundance of vaginal and penile sores. In the United States, on the other hand, the gay revolution of the 1970s brought a similar uncontrolled rise in a whole array of anal-based venereal diseases. Even without these venereal diseases, however, HIV is more easily contracted through anal intercourse because rectal walls are thin, with the blood supply close to the surface, and are designed to absorb fluids. The rectum was simply not designed for the physical trauma of intercourse, whether heterosexual or homosexual.

How easy is it to catch HIV? The probability of contracting the retrovirus remains undetermined. As noted above, HIV is naturally fragile in the environment; in addition, the potency of each donor's infective HIV antigens varies, as does the strength of the recipient's immune system and the ability of the invasive agent to find passage into the recipient's blood system. Some individuals have had unprotected anal intercourse many times with seropositive partners without contracting HIV. The vast majority of people who seek HIV testing—people who have participated in risky behaviors—prove to be uninfected. On the other hand, seroconversion often occurs after only one instance of risky behavior. Table 1 shows the relative risk levels involved in selected sexual activities.

LIVING AND DYING WITH HIV/AIDS

It may be difficult to empathize with people who have HIV/AIDS, because they undergo trauma unlike any other.[24] HIV is quite different from other disabilities, even terminal cancer, in that there is little reason for hope. While there are a few unexplained instances of protracted health, and protease inhibitors show promise of prolonging life, the overwhelming number of people with HIV will most

Table 1. Sexual Transmission of HIV: Barometer of Risk

Risk Level	Activity	Receptive	Insertive
Extremely high risk	Anal intercourse	X	—
	Anal intercourse	—	X
Very high risk	Fellatio	X	—
	Vaginal intercourse	X	—
High risk	Vaginal intercourse	—	X
	Cunnilingus	—	X
Risk	Cunnilingus	X	—
	Fellatio	—	X
No risk[a]	Kissing, mutual masturbation, massage, holding, etc.	X	X

[a]Naturally risk increases with the possibility of fluid-to-blood contact. For instance, two people who have just flossed their teeth might exchange blood in the process of kissing. Risk increases when someone with a cut or lesion on the hand masturbates someone who has cytomegalovirus or Kaposi's sarcoma lesions on or around the penis.

likely die of AIDS.[25] Although President Clinton has called for a preventive vaccine in the next decade, a cure is not yet on the horizon.[26]

A Different Kind of Dying Process

Even the process of dying is different for someone with HIV/AIDS. Because of the multitude of illnesses that occur as the immune system deteriorates, AIDS brings one of the most painful deaths known to humankind.[27] A person who is seropositive but asymptomatic sees the kind of illnesses awaiting her when she goes each month to an AIDS clinic to have a new count made of her CD_4 T-cells or whenever she attends a support group and sees people who are markedly weakened. The asymptomatic person also catches a glimpse of himself in the not-too-distant future when he visits an ailing friend on the AIDS ward of a hospital or says goodbye to someone dying in a hospice. Especially in urban areas, symptomatic people are ubiquitous and visibly remind each asymptomatic individual of the horrors that lurk just around the corner.

Acting Old Before Your Time

Although the overwhelming number of people with HIV/AIDS are young, between the ages of twenty and forty-four, many begin, as their T-cell count starts to drop, to engage in behavior that we usually associate with senior citizens. They "act old." Many scan the obituary section of the daily newspaper for the names of friends. Many also attend funerals of AIDS victims even if they did not personally know the deceased.

Persons with AIDS are forced to put their personal affairs in order. Particularly for gay people with HIV/AIDS, there may be a coming to terms with estranged family members—with fathers and brothers who have not yet accepted the homosexual orientation. People with HIV/AIDS write last wills and testaments, and they search for ways to ensure financial security for spouses or significant others. Much like senior citizens preparing for death, people with HIV/AIDS also begin to give away personal items: clothes, pictures, furniture, pets, and keepsakes. They also prepare for their own funerals: selecting grave sites and finding the limited number of funeral homes that accept the corpses of people with AIDS while neither violating confidentiality nor overcharging by insisting on unnecessary glass-sealed caskets.[28] While the young person may appear healthy as these activities take place, the CD_4 T-cell count is in decline.

Not Ready for Death

Like many others with terminal illnesses, most people with HIV/AIDS experience five stages of dying—denial, anger, bargaining, depression, and acceptance.[29] Their experiences, however, differ somewhat from those of most other dying people in at least two ways.

First, few people with HIV/AIDS seem to reach the fifth stage of dying. Even though they participate in the many rituals of dying, as old people do, the youthfulness of persons with HIV/AIDS may ultimately preclude acceptance.[30] For many of these individuals, too, the anticipation of severe pain creates a tremendous fear about the dying process that overshadows any ability to accept the approaching death. Second, someone dying of HIV/AIDS is likely to differ from someone dying of any other affliction in that he or she will move back and forth between the five stages rather than completing each one in turn.

In essence, most people with HIV/AIDS tend to experience sequentially and simultaneously the first four dimensions of dying. Denial, anger, and depression are certainly prominent during the initial period, when one has just learned of the seroconversion. Denial may manifest itself in a continuation of behaviors that were practiced prior to knowing about the infection, including unsafe sexual habits. Some people during the initial period cope with their anger by seeking out as many unsuspecting people as possible to be sexual partners. Such irresponsible behavior seems more prevalent among younger homosexual males and may well be as common today within the infected gay community as it was more than a decade ago at the start of the epidemic. The introduction of protease inhibitors, bringing hope of long-term survival and perhaps even recovery from HIV, provides an additional rationale for individuals wishing to continue unsafe sexual practices out of denial or anger. Depression always seems to accompany, and is often used to justify, behavior stemming from denial and anger. Depression, denial, and anger also seem to be factors that prevent some PLWAs from adhering to the regimen associated with protease inhibitors.

Bargaining also tends to come into play but only after some time has elapsed. The person with HIV/AIDS begins to alter past behaviors gradually, as part of an effort to strike a deal with God to change his HIV status, perhaps by engaging in unprotected sexual acts less frequently, by resisting the temptation to infect others deliberately, or by making amends with friends and loved ones. Some bargains also involve curbing drug or alcohol abuse and returning to addiction-specific support groups. Again, depression is common.

As the retrovirus progresses, or when the CD_4 T-cell count begins to drop, there is often greater acceptance that death is inevitable, but denial, anger, depression, and bargaining may return daily, even hourly. Denial may mean dreaming about cures and planning ahead for long-term relationships or vacation trips that will never occur. The promise of each new scientific advancement naturally encourages denial. There may be anger that the person will never have grandchildren, or resentment of those with higher CD_4 T-cell counts. The cost, scarcity, and strict regimen associated with protease inhibitors preclude their success with many people with HIV/AIDS, and this becomes another avenue for anger. There may also be hatred of past lovers who, fearful of contracting HIV/AIDS, have abandoned the sufferer.

The bargaining process involves a long-term struggle, with a variety of "deals" offered in return for staying alive and healthy a bit longer. Many seropositive individuals who were once self-centered or even selfish now volunteer to help AIDS-related groups and causes. Some PLWAs begin to devote more time to the needs of neighbors, friends, and family members. Still others become religious, in many instances for the first time in their lives.

A Roller Coaster of Emotions and Fears

During the prolonged period of reasonably good health characteristic of the asymptomatic stage, people often go from one emotional extreme to another as they grapple with the fear of dying. They watch the slow but inevitable decline in CD_4 T-cells. When therapy includes the use of protease inhibitors, asymptomatic persons hope that the treatment will be effective but also know that this is not always the case. They are also painfully aware of the consequences of not strictly adhering each day to the regimen associated with the protease inhibitors. They begin to take stock of the number of good days and months and begin to realize that bad days and months certainly lie ahead.

Once AIDS symptoms begin to appear, or when the CD_4 T-cell count drops below 200, life becomes both physically and emotionally unpredictable. People may feel near death one month, go into temporary remission, and be reasonably healthy again the next month—or at least sufficiently healthy to return to work. The good days and months dwindle in number and quality, however.

DEMOGRAPHICS OF HIV/AIDS

How many Americans have HIV? Estimates range from about 1 million to well over 5 million people.[31] The question cannot be answered precisely for three reasons. First, an exact answer would necessitate testing everyone for the presence of HIV antibodies every ninety days because antibodies are not detectable during most of the acute HIV stage. The American public health system is not prepared to test over 265 million people four times a year for a total of more than one billion people annually.

Second, difficulties in determining the number of people who have HIV stem from the fact that the vast majority of these people are unaware of their condition. They are asymptomatic and, for reasons explained above, will most likely remain so for about ten years after infection. As long as apparent health conditions do not arouse concern, most people who are seropositive feel no urgent need to arrange for testing.

The third factor preventing an exact count of people with HIV has to do with the anonymous testing procedures that have been adopted in every state. Anonymous positive test results are not reported for at least three reasons. First, many states prohibit the reporting of anonymous HIV test results. The rationale is that by keeping the process and results completely secret, the state can encourage people to be tested. Second, persons whose test results are positive frequently seek retesting in an effort to double-check (or even triple-check) the horrific findings. The inclusion of anonymous test results would involve an unknown amount of duplication. Third, expanding the official count to encompass anonymous positive HIV test results would preclude effective epidemiological tracking. The public health system would not know when to shift specific individuals on the HIV list to the list of those with full-blown AIDS. Similarly, there would be no way of knowing when to shift specific persons onto the roll of people who have died of AIDS.[32] It is important to have such information if we are to gain a more thorough understanding of the epidemic's dynamics.

Several states have begun to permit confidential HIV testing, where the person's name is affixed to test results. Table 2 shows the states that now report such test findings. It is important to note that individuals seeking testing in these states still have options; only *confidential* test results, and not *anonymous* test results, are reported. It is also important to note that the three states with over 45 percent of all AIDS cases—New York, California, and Florida—still do not report positive HIV test results.

We are better able to estimate the number of people with AIDS. Demographic data suggest three fundamental trends. First, the number of PLWAs continues to

Table 2. States That Report Confidential HIV Testing Results

State	Date Initiated HIV Reporting	State	Date Initiated HIV Reporting
Alabama	Jan. 1988	North Carolina	Feb. 1990
Arizona	Jan. 1987	North Dakota	Jan. 1988
Arkansas	July 1989	Ohio	June 1990
Colorado	Nov. 1985	Oklahoma	June 1988
Connecticut[a]	July 1992	Oregon[b]	Sept. 1988
Idaho	June 1986	South Carolina	Feb. 1986
Indiana	July 1988	South Dakota	Jan. 1988
Louisiana	Feb. 1993	Tennessee	Jan. 1992
Michigan	April 1992	Texas[a]	Feb. 1994
Minnesota	Oct. 1985	Utah	April 1989
Mississippi	Aug. 1988	Virginia	July 1989
Missouri	Oct. 1987	West Virginia	Jan. 1989
Nebraska	Sept. 1995	Wisconsin	Nov. 1985
Nevada	Feb. 1992	Wyoming	June 1989
New Jersey	Jan. 1992		

[a]Confidential testing only for pediatric cases. [b]Confidential testing only for children less than 6.
Source: Centers for Disease Control and Prevention. *HIV/AIDS Surveillance Report* 9:1 (1997): 26, table 22.

escalate exponentially. Since the early 1980s, approximately 700,000 Americans have developed full-blown AIDS. The number of PLWAs in this country increased by 25 percent in 1993 and by another 20 percent in 1994. With approximately one new case reported every 11.5 minutes in this country, more than 130 Americans will be diagnosed with AIDS before this day is over. As you read this book, keep in mind that one American will die of AIDS about every eight minutes throughout the day.

The second trend is that members of all groups in society are vulnerable, regardless of ethnicity and gender. Currently 90 percent of PLWAs are of working age, and 75 percent of them are in the prime working ages of twenty-five to forty-four. Moreover, AIDS is the number one cause of death for both men and women between the ages of twenty and forty-four.

The third demographic trend indicates that AIDS has struck in every region of the country, regardless of whether the location is urban or rural in nature. Since the early 1980s, the AIDS epidemic in America has killed about as many people as those who live in Cincinnati, Ohio. New York, Los Angeles, and San Francisco together still account for about one-third of all AIDS cases. The epidemic nevertheless affects every major metropolitan area, for an average of about 6,000 AIDS cases per city.

FRAMEWORK FOR ANALYSIS

HIV is a retrovirus that attacks and destroys the body's immune system over a period of time ranging from just a few years to well over a decade. By destroying the immune system, HIV promotes the onslaught of AIDS. Fluid-to-blood contact is required for transmission of the HIV retrovirus. The social stigma attached to the epidemic, the relatively young age of most people within the HIV spectrum, and the painful and devastating syndrome of opportunistic infections, diseases, and cancers—all make living with HIV and dying of AIDS a most excruciating process. People of every ethnicity and both genders are equally susceptible to HIV if they engage in risky behaviors. HIV/AIDS affects primarily people of working age. At least until they are diagnosed, most people within the HIV spectrum are holding jobs and pursuing careers. We must understand the background characteristics and dynamics of HIV/AIDS before we can profitably examine its effects on the workplace.

This book looks at workplace ramifications of HIV/AIDS in the public service and specifically in local government. I chose the municipal workplace because it collectively employs the largest group of workers in the United States. My research examined four dimensions of the problem. The first dimension is legal constraints on ways of coping with HIV/AIDS in the workforce. The second dimension is attitudes toward seropositive job applicants and employees. The focus here is on the views of local government practitioners on the general topic of HIV/AIDS, the selection and screening of employees, confidentiality of employee health status, citizen contact with employees in the HIV spectrum, reasonable accommodations, and undue hardship. The third dimension is the appropriate response by local governments to the epidemic in their workplaces. Included here are concerns about the adoption of HIV/AIDS plans and various ways of assisting the employee and job applicant with HIV/AIDS. The fourth dimension relates to the level of preparedness within local government and involves factors such as form of government, community characteristics, personal backgrounds of practitioners, and the organizational experiences city halls have gained in managing previous HIV/AIDS-related situations.

Preparedness entails having some sort of plan or a set of strategies in place to respond to the HIV/AIDS epidemic in the workforce. As with any other type of public emergency, the development of a plan of action must precede any testing of the plan's usefulness. Unfortunately it remains true today, as when the first edition of this book was written, that most local government officials are only beginning to grasp the direct effect of the HIV/AIDS epidemic on their workforce. Consequently many officials are only just beginning to talk about a plan of action. I have therefore deliberately focused on issues and questions surrounding the development of responsive strategies and not on the effectiveness of those plans once they are in place. Unfortunately it is too soon to gauge the impact of local government

HIV/AIDS plans. My aim in these pages is not only to facilitate understanding of the dynamics of workforce management in the age of AIDS but also to help frame questions for further research into ways of coping with the crisis that the HIV/AIDS epidemic presents to the public service.

Chapter 2, "HIV/AIDS, Public Policy, and the Public Service," argues that the epidemic presents a crisis to public agencies. Chapter 3, "HIV/AIDS and the Law," delineates HIV/AIDS-related workplace responsibilities of both public and private employers. Here the focus is much more on the application of the Americans with Disabilities Act (ADA) and the Rehabilitation (Rehab) Act than was the case in the first edition of the book. Chapter 4, "Attitudes toward HIV/AIDS in the Workplace," analyzes the views of local government officials about the rights of employees and job applicants who are in the HIV spectrum. Chapter 5, "Workplace Policies and Procedures," investigates the degree to which HIV/AIDS policies and practices have been initiated by local governments throughout the United States. It also looks at the forces that contribute to local government preparedness in the workplace. Both chapters 4 and 5 are based on new survey data. Chapter 6, "HIV/AIDS and the Public Service: The Crisis Revisited," summarizes the findings and offers recommendations as to how we might improve the level of preparedness of municipalities.

2

HIV/AIDS, Public Policy, and the Public Service

THE CONSEQUENCES OF the HIV retrovirus are most conspicuous on the external side of bureaucracy, where it affects both the level of services and the manner in which those services are delivered. HIV/AIDS affects service delivery, however, primarily because of actions taken on the internal side of bureaucracy, where hiring decisions are made and personnel policies and practices are created for the workplace. By addressing the internal, workforce-related concerns emanating from the HIV/AIDS epidemic, government may be better able to address issues of service delivery. This chapter consider⸱ the impact of HIV/AIDS on public policy, the workplace, and especially the public sector workplace.

THE IMPACT OF HIV/AIDS ON PUBLIC POLICY

The relationship between HIV/AIDS and public policy is unique. Although, as Scott Burris reminds us, "HIV is not unique among diseases in provoking controversy," HIV/AIDS differs from other diseases with social impacts in being a truly *public* epidemic with *public* ramifications.[1] Rheumatoid arthritis or cancer, for instance, is not "public" in the same sense as HIV/AIDS, because, today, neither disease potentially endangers all individuals of working age, and consequently, neither threatens the well-being of the American economic and social infrastructures.

Nor do most contagious diseases pose a public threat in the same way as HIV/AIDS.[2] Because the epidemic concentrated initially in the gay community, the stigma associated with it is very different from that associated with other communicable diseases such as chlamydia or tuberculosis.[3] In addition, non-AIDS-related contagious diseases can be managed through standard public health procedures: epidemiological tracking, dissemination of tracking-based information, mass testing and inoculation, and, if necessary, forced isolation and quarantine. In contrast, how could society quarantine the millions of people in this country who are probably HIV positive? And for what epidemiological reasons? How could society restrict the social behaviors of every person with HIV/AIDS? While other contagions create local crises at times, and media attention generates some national concern, the resulting public problems are far less complex and much easier to manage than those created by HIV/AIDS.

15

Culture and Policy

The distinctive nature of HIV/AIDS may well require unique public policy responses. But responses are often limited by the way in which people define problems as well as by the manner and extent to which they permit government to find solutions. In the case of HIV/AIDS, society's generalized attitudes and belief systems—its social and political culture—bear a particularly close relationship to policy responses. As in every other nation, national values affect the way in which HIV/AIDS is defined and understood. Moreover, the cultural-political definition of HIV/AIDS has an impact on government's ability to take action and to lead the way in addressing all facets of this crisis.

In the United States, HIV/AIDS is understood through two fundamental cultural values. The first is homophobia. From the very outset, HIV/AIDS was more closely associated with male homosexuals than with any other segment of American society. Scientists initially dubbed the disease "GRID," for Gay-Related Immune Deficiency, because the first identified cases were homosexual men. In the early 1980s, the gay community often called the disease "gay cancer." Even today, when American heterosexual men and women are contracting the retrovirus in ever-increasing numbers, two-thirds of all Americans with AIDS are either homosexual or bisexual men.[4]

Second, a commitment to individual rights influences the way in which Americans understand HIV/AIDS. This commitment is especially pertinent for the gay community, which, in some areas of the United States, during the 1970s fought for and won some basic civil rights that other Americans take for granted.[5] Municipal ordinances were enacted to prohibit discrimination against homosexuals in housing, jobs, and access to public facilities.[6] The legal recognition of homosexual ghettos, nightclubs, and bathhouses, as well as local government–embraced celebrations like San Francisco's "Gay Freedom Day," helped increase the self-esteem and political strength of gay people in many urban areas. The gay community, therefore, viewed the epidemic and public response to it initially with mistrust. HIV/AIDS was seen as a potential weapon that conservative groups could use to deprive gay Americans of the many civil rights that they had won in the 1970s. To a great extent, the views held by gay Americans today remain unchanged.[7]

The Role of Government

As Randy Shilts observed, "AIDS did not just happen to America—it was allowed to happen by an array of institutions all of which failed to perform their appropriate tasks to safeguard the public health."[8] In short, social and cultural norms have affected the manner in which government, and government-dependent organizations, have responded to the HIV/AIDS crisis.[9]

The initial assumption that HIV/AIDS was a gay disease meant that the policy response was more desultory than it might have been if a greater number of people in mainstream heterosexual society had been known to be at risk.[10] Especially in the early stages of the epidemic, government indecisiveness may be interpreted in a variety of ways. The federal government, for instance, was unwilling to designate the outbreak of HIV/AIDS an epidemic although several hundred cases of AIDS had already been reported by the end of 1981. One explanation might be a lack of understanding; most politicians were probably not aware of the magnitude of the problem until prominent people in society died in the late 1980s.

But a more proactive and aggressive response might also have resulted in adverse political consequences for key national leaders. How could politicians such as Jesse Helms and Strom Thurmond, who opposed homosexuality, acknowledge the need to combat a disease that seemed confined to the gay community? Certainly by doing so they would have risked alienating conservative voters and like-minded political action committees. Many other elected officials throughout the United States probably also preferred to distance themselves from an infectious agent that highlighted sociocultural deviance and prejudice as it killed people.[11]

Many Red Cross and public health officials were similarly ambivalent about designating HIV/AIDS as an epidemic.[12] They shared fears of adverse consequences, some of which related to the blood industry. In the early 1980s, the nation's blood supply depended heavily on the contributions of many civic-minded gay men as well as on blood sold by the poor and homeless. Public health officials feared that an alarmed public might enact laws designed to prohibit homosexuals from contributing to blood banks and might therefore drastically reduce the nation's blood supply.

The scientific community, heavily subsidized by the federal government, was also in a quandary about the retrovirus's homosexual overtones.[13] Younger researchers at the CDC, and at many research universities across the nation, were eager to forge ahead with possibly the greatest epidemiological investigation of their careers. But mentors and supervisors restrained some from spending exorbitant amounts of time pursuing answers to a "gay disease." Successful careers and reputations, they were instructed, could not be built on such an endeavor. The same attitude was reflected in the National Institutes of Health's decision in the early 1980s to withhold funding from projects that proposed to study gay-related diseases. As Shilts observed, the few scientists who chose to search for a cure to AIDS "found themselves not only struggling against a baffling disease but against the indifference of science, government, and public health officials."[14]

The fact that HIV/AIDS was defined as an attack on the civil liberties of homosexuals also profoundly limited the government's response.[15] Gay activists successfully fought public health officials' attempts to close down bathhouses, which were regarded as places to exercise the constitutional right of free association. Because the promiscuous sexual behavior associated with bathhouses was not halted, the retrovirus spread rapidly among members of the gay community.

And because HIV/AIDS was defined in terms of two conflicting norms, civil rights and homophobia, public health officials did not adopt basic public health strategies designed to control epidemics and protect the public health.[16] The social stigma attached to being HIV positive impeded serious discussions about mass HIV antibody blood testing. Gay leaders argued that the chances of losing employment, housing, and health insurance—as a result of having a "gay disease"—were simply too great to institute large-scale screening. While traditional confinement would not prevent the retrovirus from spreading, restricting the sexual activities of its victims might reduce the number of people who would unknowingly contract it.[17] Regardless of the need to control the epidemic's spread, civil libertarians and gay activists opposed the use of any quarantine strategy as diminishing the rights and status of individuals with HIV/AIDS.

It would be misleading to suggest that the American political culture has exerted no positive effects on government's efforts to respond to this crisis. Even homophobia was helpful initially in pointing American epidemiologists and public health officials in the right direction to track the retrovirus. As Shilts noted, the disease's homosexual link was missed completely by European scientists and public health officials, who are less culturally preoccupied with alternative lifestyles and practices.

Furthermore, because HIV/AIDS was defined in terms of civil rights, funding levels were disproportionately higher than those for research on other diseases, like breast, prostate, and lung cancers, which tend to affect greater numbers of people. The federal government spends approximately $6 billion annually, more than all other nations combined, on HIV/AIDS activities across numerous departments and independent agencies.[18] The civil rights aspect also helps account for the amount of funding that finds its way into a variety of nonresearch categories, from housing subsidies to emergency cash for food and pharmaceuticals.[19] Perhaps primarily for this reason, the HIV/AIDS crisis intervention systems of other nations, including telephone hot lines and case management, cannot compare in quality or quantity to the services available in the United States.

Yet American culture slows progress in many of the battles against the HIV retrovirus.[20] At the core, HIV/AIDS is creating a policy crisis over attempts to balance two constitutional imperatives: the need to protect the health and safety of the public and the need to protect the civil rights of individuals with HIV/AIDS in all facets of daily life. The policy crisis is pitting well-intentioned groups concerned about the civil liberties of those in the HIV spectrum against equally well-intentioned groups with concerns about the rights of uninfected individuals.[21] Anxiety about the disease also fuels extremist elements in society; the Lyndon LaRouche–sponsored "Prevent AIDS Now Initiative Committee" (PANIC), for example, in 1986 unsuccessfully sought California voters' approval for mass testing and quarantining of citizens in the HIV spectrum.[22]

It is as important and difficult to resolve the policy crisis as it is to find a cure for the retrovirus. And given the constitutional issues involved, it is absolutely essential that appropriate policy choices be made. For instance, there is danger in erring on the side of "doing." As one observer cogently remarked, "Policies dominated by overreaction threaten to build walls around sick people and victimize them, and even the most robust democracy may not be strong enough to withstand such divisive forces."[23] Even though PANIC's scheme was rejected by the majority of California voters, there was enough support to place it on the ballot. Would similar proposals be defeated in every state or a second time in California? There is no guarantee that voters in a democracy will respond rationally to the issues presented to them.

Yet equally dangerous is the act of erring on the side of indecision. The public needs to understand quite thoroughly the HIV disease and all of its ramifications: the nature and pattern of the epidemic, current and projected expenses relevant to treatment and finding a cure, and the incumbent legal, administrative, and workplace issues.[24] Because adequate precautions are needed for both noninfected and seropositive citizens, policymakers must experiment and "engage in extraordinary efforts to initiate large and non-incremental change."[25] Tough or not, choices about the allocation of limited resources must be made.

We must not become paralyzed either by the fear of the retrovirus or the fear of overreaction in responding to HIV/AIDS. Political correctness, whatever its orientation, must not dictate society's course of action. The differences between potentially reactive and proactive strategies are not always clear-cut. In view of the nature of this epidemic, doing nothing about HIV/AIDS and its consequences is the worst choice possible.

HIV/AIDS IN THE WORKPLACE

Given the modes of HIV transmission, why is a discussion about HIV/AIDS and the workplace needed? Although the overwhelming majority of people with HIV/AIDS are probably members of the *workforce,* does that fact alone make the epidemic a *workplace* issue?[26] Certainly most workplaces are not the source of HIV transmission; even workplaces with a very high risk of fluids-to-blood contact, such as hospital emergency rooms and trauma centers, pose little threat to workers and citizens alike as long as regulations of the Occupational Safety and Health Administration (OSHA) regarding blood-borne pathogens are followed strictly. Very few employees in higher-risk settings, particularly the health care fields (see table 3), have acquired HIV/AIDS through workplace activities. Whether we are discussing the trauma center of Los Angeles County Hospital, the sanitation department of New York City, the Chicago Fire Department, or the budget office for the city of Miami, the workplace is perhaps the safest area of personal interaction with the least risk of contagion. So why is HIV/AIDS a workplace issue?

First, the workplace rights of people with HIV/AIDS are protected by law. As

Table 3. Health Care Workers with Documented and Possible Occupationally
Acquired AIDS/HIV Infection, by Occupation, Reported Through June 1997,
United States

Occupation	Documented Cases[a]	Possible Casesb
Dental worker, including dentists	—	7
Embalmer/morgue technician	—	2
Emergency medical technician/paramedic	—	10
Health aide/attendant	1	12
Housekeeper/maintenance worker	1	7
Laboratory technician, clinical	16	16
Laboratory technician, nonclinical	3	1
Nurse	21	29
Physician, nonsurgical	6	10
Physician, surgical	—	6
Respiratory therapist	1	2
Technician, dialysis	1	3
Technician, surgical	2	2
Technician/therapist, other than those listed above	—	5
Other health care occupations	—	2
Total	52	114

Note: Health care workers are defined as those persons, including students and trainees, who have worked in a health care, clinical, or HIV laboratory setting at any time since 1978.

[a]Health care workers who had documented HIV seroconversion after occupational exposure or had other laboratory evidence of occupational infection: 44 had percutaneous exposure, 5 had mucocutaneous exposure, 1 had both percutaneous and mucocutaneous exposures, and 1 had an unknown route of exposure. Forty-six exposures were to blood from an HIV-infected person, 1 to visibly bloody fluid, 1 to an unspecified fluid, and 3 to concentrated virus in a laboratory. Twenty-four of these health care workers developed AIDS.

[b]These health care workers have been investigated and are without identifiable behavioral or transfusion risks; each reported percutaneous or mucocutaneous occupational exposures to blood or body fluids, or to laboratory solutions containing HIV, but HIV seroconversion specifically resulting from an occupational exposure was not documented.

Source: Centers for Disease Control and Prevention, *HIV/AIDS Surveillance Report* 9:1 (1997): 15, table 11.

we will see in Chapter 3, the Rehabilitation Act and the Americans with Disabilities Act (ADA) protect employees and job applicants with HIV/AIDS from discriminatory acts at the workplace. Because of the retrovirus, then, laws place additional burdens on management and its budget.

Second, and more important, fear makes HIV/AIDS a workplace issue.[27] Fear transcends the behavior of infected and noninfected employees alike and reaches supervisors and employers of the work organization. Fear of HIV/AIDS affects both worker morale and workplace productivity.

Employees with HIV/AIDS carry with them the fear of dying from a combination of horrific infections and illnesses. As we saw in Chapter 1, they live with constant and varied reminders of the agonies that they will most likely experience in a relatively short period of time. They also live with the stigma of having HIV/AIDS and may therefore feel that they must hide their fears as well as their declining health. Consequently the ability of employees with HIV/AIDS to do their jobs in a satisfactory manner may be challenged by physical and emotional disorders and also by disruptions that result from constant shifts in physical and psychological well-being. The "bad days" that people with HIV/AIDS experience may translate into a corresponding number of less productive days at the workplace. HIV/AIDS also affects the workplace, then, by making good employees look and act bad.

Fears of noninfected employees and supervisors generally center around the issue of contagion. Certainly most workers understand that unsafe sexual practices and intravenous drug use are the primary modes of transmission. But medicine is an imprecise science, and the remote possibility that one worker with cuts or open sores on his hands will transmit HIV to another worker with similar cuts or open sores remains in the 1990s a worrisome proposition to many rational individuals. Although epidemiologists insist that casual contact with HIV infected individuals is safe, we know that even dentists today take the precaution of wearing surgical gloves and goggles for protection from HIV/AIDS.[28] People sitting in the dentist chair often do not notice that dentists take such precautions because detailed procedures normally involve contact with blood.

The anxiety of uncertainty engenders suspicion and fears about HIV/AIDS in the work space as it does elsewhere in society. This is the most dangerous kind of fear—the fear that we may be wrong. As Judith Wilson Ross reminds us, "We have spent our lives in a culture in which infectious disease does not represent a significant threat and thus we had consigned living in fear of life-threatening contagious diseases to the pages of history books."[29] The need of present generations to reexamine faith in the certainty of science, coupled with the fact that people cannot choose coworkers and supervisors, causes much doubt and fear about routine human interactions at work. This, too, is a workplace ramification of HIV/AIDS.

Anxiety about HIV infection gives many employees and supervisors common ground on which to stand. But workplace managers are also concerned about margins of profit or, in the public sector, about financial management and productivity.

Administrators are noticing three general areas of added expense: (1) productivity costs, (2) health care benefit costs, and (3) the cost of compliance with government regulations and procedures. Added expense is another reason why HIV/AIDS is a workplace issue.

How much will the epidemic cost workplace organizations? The answer varies, depending on several factors. Seropositive individuals have different needs, depending on the particular detectable stages of the disease: asymptomatic, persistent generalized lymphadenopathy, or full-blown AIDS. Once a person's CD_4 T-cell count has dropped sufficiently to allow for the introduction of AIDS-related opportunistic infections and diseases, costs will reflect the particular symptoms and illnesses experienced.

For instance, the average annual cost of trimethopic-sulfurmethoxazole, a drug used to treat *pneumocystis carinii* pneumonia and *toxoplasma gondii* is only $400.[30] The average annual cost for 3200 milligrams daily of acyclovir, used in the treatment of cytomegalovirus (CMV)/herpes, is about $5,115.[31] The average annual cost of 600 milligram daily doses of azidothymidine (AZT) and didanosine (ddI), two of the primary antiviral drugs, is approximately $8,000 for each. Newer antiretroviral protease inhibitors, such as sequinavir and ritonavir, cost approximately $10,000 each year.

Typically someone with AIDS may take both AZT and ddI, perhaps as many as five other experimental antiviral drugs, like Remune and Vistide, and an assortment of herbs, vitamins, and other concoctions.[32] Protease inhibitors are typically taken in "cocktail" form with at least two other antiviral drugs, AZT, ddI, zalcitabine (ddC), stavudine (d4T), or lamivudine (3TC). In many instances, seropositive individuals will begin taking antiviral drugs, nutrient supplements, and protease inhibitors during the asymptomatic stage in an effort to delay as long as possible the onslaught of opportunistic illnesses and AIDS-related cancers.

Costs also vary according to the place of treatment and the date when treatment begins. Individuals with HIV/AIDS who live in larger and more urban locations—settings that have not only a critical mass of people with HIV/AIDS but also a decade or more of experience in dealing with the retrovirus—are able to minimize costs much more easily than people within the HIV spectrum who live in more rural and isolated communities.[33] If someone begins treatment earlier in the progression of the HIV retrovirus, especially at the asymptomatic stage, then total pharmaceutical costs tend to be higher, while costs for hospitalization may be somewhat delayed and perhaps even lessened. For someone who defers treatment, the cost of hospitalization will probably be much higher and more immediate, while pharmaceutical costs may be lower ultimately because of an abbreviated life span. According to a Kaiser Permanente study made in northern California, the average person with full-blown AIDS experiences 3.5 hospitalizations, with each visit lasting approximately forty days.[34] Officials in the CDC estimate that the average an-

Table 4. Estimated Workplace Cost of HIV/AIDS per Seropositive Employee: Self-Insured Municipalities

Year	Health Condition	Health Care Cost	Sick Days[a] Cost/No. (#)	Reasonable Accommodation	Life Insurance	Total Cost
99	HIV+	$ 7,500	$ 923.12 (8)	$ 0	$—	$ 8,423.12
00	HIV+	7,500	576.95 (5)	0	—	8,076.95
01	HIV+	7,500	576.95 (5)	0	—	8,076.95
02	HIV+	7,500	576.95 (5)	100	—	8,176.95
03	HIV+	7,500	576.95 (5)	100	—	8,176.95
04	HIV+	7,500	576.95 (5)	100	—	8,176.95
05	HIV+	7,500	576.95 (5)	100	—	8,176.95
06	HIV+	7,500	576.95 (5)	100	—	8,176.95
07	HIV+	7,500	576.95 (5)	100	—	8,176.95
08	PGL	7,500	1,153.90 (10)	500	—	9,153.90
09	PGL	7,500	1,730.85 (15)	500	—	9,730.85
10	AIDS	28,725	2,884.75 (25)	1,000	—	32,609.75
11	Death	28,725	$ 4,615.60 (40)	1,000	50,000	84,340.60
Total		$139,950	$15,923.82	$3,600	$50,000	$209,473.82

Note: PGL = persistent generalized lymphadenopathy.
[a] Includes 20 percent non–health care fringe benefits.
Source: Adapted from Jack P. DeSario, Sue R. Faerman, and James D. Slack, *Local Government Information and Training Needs in the 21st Century* (Westport, CT: Quorum Books, 1994), 34. Further modifications based on suggestions from Irene S. Rubin, Northern Illinois University, Sylvester Murray, Cleveland State University, and Herbert V. Kaighan, senior vice president of Godwins, Booke and Dickenson.

nual health care cost is $15,000 for someone who is experiencing effects up through the PGL stage and $45,000 for someone who has AIDS.[35]

Yet these estimates do not accurately reflect all costs incurred in the workplace. Total expenditures will depend on a number of factors, including the percentage of health care costs covered by the group insurance, ceilings on health care coverage, whether the organization is self-insured, the amount of group life insurance, the forms of accommodation that are feasible and reasonable, and the salary and life span of the seropositive employee.

Such disparate factors make for a complex picture, as the two examples in tables 4 and 5 suggest. Table 4 offers an understated, conservative estimate of workplace costs for a self-insured municipality.[36] The figures reflect the following assumptions. First, the employee with HIV will live for thirteen years. In this scenario, he or she is infected with HIV on January 1, 1999, and will die of AIDS on December 31, 2011. The person will spend the first nine years in the asymptomatic stage. The final four years will be marked by PGL and full-blown AIDS. Second, like many other people with HIV/AIDS, the employee will be able to work well into the year of death. Third, the cost of reasonable accommodations, which will be discussed thoroughly in Chapter 3, will increase as the person progresses through the stages of the disease. Reasonable accommodations may encompass flextime, additional sick days, job relocation, and working at home. Figures for the cost of reasonable accommodations are based on estimates provided by the Job Accommodation Network.[37] Fourth, the person earns an annual salary of $25,000, which means that one sick day costs the employer $96.16. Fifth, 75 percent of all health care costs are picked up by the employer through self-insurance. Finally, the employer agrees to pay $50,000 in the form of life insurance.

Table 5 shows the cost for municipalities with group health care and life insurance packages. The same background assumptions apply here as in table 4, except that the employer now pays only a flat premium for both health care and life insurance packages. The premiums reflect averages among municipalities in southern California and include a 12 percent rate of increase that has been fairly constant for the past decade.[38]

The estimates in table 5, like those in table 4, are understated. In addition, they do not take into consideration the distinct possibility of rate increases based on utilization. This possibility, which typically affects smaller municipalities, means that the estimates found in table 5 are perhaps slightly more conservative (understated) than those in table 4.[39]

As the numbers in table 4 and table 5 indicate, each workplace will experience at least four cost-related ramifications of HIV/AIDS. First, every employee within the HIV spectrum will cost the self-insured work organization almost $210,000. For organizations with insurance packages, the costs drop to about $136,000. Given that the employer will have to pay insurance premiums regardless of utilization, the actual cost for a seropositive employee drops to about $22,000. Even though these expenses vary somewhat in different regions, the rate of increase will be relatively constant from year to year for the life of the employee.

Second, the total cost of sick days will be significant for each workplace and in some regions may match the cost of hiring one additional part-time staff member (at $15,000) for at least one full year. Third, expenses associated with reasonable accommodations will not be as great as anticipated by many managers. Contrary to management's biggest fear, reasonable accommodation may actually represent the least burdensome cost to the work organization.

Fourth, the largest workplace expenditure will be providing health care: over two-thirds of all costs incurred by self-insured municipalities and nearly 85 percent of the workplace-related costs for municipalities with health care packages. It is also important to remember that the costs of health care are increasing because of many

Table 5. Estimated Workplace Cost of HIV/AIDS per Seropositive Employee: Municipalities with Group Health and Life Insurance Packages

Year	Health Condition	Health Care Cost	Sick Days[a] Cost/No. (#)	Reasonable Accommodation	Life Insurance	Total Cost
99	HIV+	$ 4,100	$ 923.12 (8)	$ 0	$ 150	$ 5,173.12
00	HIV+	4,592	576.95 (5)	0	150	5,318.95
01	HIV+	5,143	576.95 (5)	0	150	5,869.95
02	HIV+	5,760	576.95 (5)	100	150	6,586.95
03	HIV+	6,451	576.95 (5)	100	150	7,277.95
04	HIV+	7,225	576.95 (5)	100	150	8,051.95
05	HIV+	8,092	576.95 (5)	100	150	8,918.95
06	HIV+	9,063	576.95 (5)	100	150	9,889.95
07	HIV+	10,151	576.95 (5)	100	150	10,977.95
08	PGL	11,369	1,153.90 (10)	500	150	13,172.90
09	PGL	12,733	1,730.85 (15)	500	150	15,113.85
10	AIDS	14,261	2,884.75 (25)	1,000	150	18,295.75
11	Death	15,972	4,615.60 (40)	1,000	150	21,737.60
Total		$114,912	$15,923.82	$3,600	$1,950	$136,385.82

Note: PGL = persistent generalized lymphadenopathy.

[a] Includes 20 percent non–health care fringe benefits.

Source: Adapted from Jack P. DeSario, Sue R. Faerman, and James D. Slack, *Local Government Information and Training Needs in the 21st Century* (Westport, CT: Quorum Books, 1994), 34. Further modifications were made using suggestions from Irene Rubin, Northern Illinois University, Sylvester Murray, Cleveland State University, and Herbert V. Kaighan, senior vice president of Godwins, Booke and Dickenson.

factors, including HIV/AIDS, regardless of whether the organization employs someone who is seropositive.

Throughout the 1980s and early 1990s, many employers attempted to cap, or place a special ceiling on, the amount of health benefits that employees with HIV/ AIDS could receive. This step was taken to avoid rate increases due to perceived overutilization. The typical cap was $5,000 in any one year and $10,000 total for HIV/AIDS, a practice that was permitted by the courts under the 1974 Employee Retirement Income Security Act (ERISA).[40] With the passage of the ADA, however, federal courts as well as the Equal Employment Opportunity Commission (EEOC) have determined that employers cannot use caps to discriminate among diseases covered through workplace insurance.[41] Workplace protections mandated by the ADA, in essence, supersede managerial discretions made available by ERISA. It therefore appears that health care for employees with HIV/AIDS will be financed by management and the work organization, either through self-in-surance or by securing insurance packages.

Two exogenous factors make management's burden of financing health care for employees within the HIV spectrum even greater. First, people with HIV/AIDS are typically unable to secure individual health insurance and must therefore rely on coverage at the workplace. Second, federal and state governments provide mini-mal health care assistance to PLWAs and only when they are indigent. While the person is able to work, therefore, government does little to lessen the financial re-sponsibilities of management.

Insurance companies make it increasingly difficult for people with HIV/AIDS to get individual health and life coverage, because greater costs associated with the retrovirus result in fewer profits. To compensate, many companies have raised premium rates and have added clauses specifying that HIV/AIDS as a preexisting condition disqualifies the person from coverage.[42] Some insurance companies also refuse to cover people who have taken HIV antibody blood tests and who are there-fore suspected of being within the HIV spectrum.[43] Such unlawful actions are taken without having the actual evidence of a preexisting HIV condition.[44]

Most insurance companies discriminate against people with HIV/AIDS and do so within the boundaries of the law. A New York court of appeals, for instance, was the first to rule that insurance companies conducting business in that state are not compelled by state regulations to underwrite health insurance policies for indi-viduals in the HIV spectrum. According to the New York court, an insurance com-pany is free to "select its risks."[45] Insurance companies are permitted to make this assumption in every state.

Federal and state governments continue to provide only marginal assistance to people with HIV/AIDS who are not their own employees and thus add to manage-ment's burden to provide health care insurance. As of 1997, less than 10 percent of federal HIV/AIDS funding went for cash assistance. Medicaid, a state program with matching funds from the federal government to pay the medical expenses of dependent and indigent individuals, is currently providing most of the public assis-tance for HIV/AIDS health care costs. The Ryan White Comprehensive AIDS Re-sources Emergency (CARE) Act of 1990 provides some funding for health care and pharmaceuticals, as well as for food and shelter, but it does so for individuals with HIV/AIDS only when they fall into the most desperate financial condition. The U.S. Department of Housing and Urban Development provides "Housing Opportu-nities for People with AIDS" (HOPWA) funds for short-term rent, mortgage, and utility payments in an effort to minimize homelessness for persons within the HIV spectrum.[46] Some federal government assistance is also available through the Title II Disability Insurance Benefit Program for persons who are too sick to keep their jobs.

The various states also provide some marginal assistance to AIDS patients. Many have "general relief" programs for indigents who are ineligible for Medicaid.

Rhode Island has enacted catastrophic health insurance legislation to cover costly and unexpected illnesses, including AIDS. California and New York provide in-home health care for PLWAs who are too weak to care for themselves and cannot afford to hire a nurse. Many states have also developed pharmaceutical programs and lotteries to assist in covering the cost of the antiviral drugs.[47]

HIV/AIDS is a workplace issue not just because it has the ability to affect the vast majority of people in the American workforce but also because (1) federal laws make it one, (2) fears of infected and noninfected coworkers make it so, and (3) concerns about current and future financing of employee health care and other workplace costs place it among employers' operating expenses. Because HIV/AIDS can adversely affect the morale and productivity of infected and noninfected workers alike, as well as influencing the financial condition of the organization, the workplace ramifications of HIV/AIDS will undoubtedly take center stage as both the private and public sectors enter the twenty-first century.

THE IMPACT OF HIV/AIDS ON THE PUBLIC SERVICE

In addition to its impact on the workplace in general, the HIV/AIDS epidemic poses a special crisis for the public service.[48] The consequences of the retrovirus can be seen most readily on the external side of public administration, in the delivery of services to the citizenry. But bureaucratic concern stems primarily from the epidemic's impact on its internal side. This dimension of bureaucracy entails recruitment, promotion, and retention decisions and determination of the policies and attitudes that formally and informally regulate behavior throughout the entire organization. Such internal, human resource management (HRM) practices obviously bear on the nature of the workforce and also help shape bureaucracy's external relationship with the citizenry. It is therefore important to investigate the internal dimensions of bureaucracy.

The External Side of Bureaucracy

Government, according to Woodrow Wilson, serves as the "instrument of humanity, of social betterment."[49] This philosophy lies at the heart of bureaucracy's external responsibilities to the public and can be applied to liberal and conservative politics alike. The belief that government should strive to improve the quality of life for the citizenry is evident in most public actions taken throughout American history. Examples might include the Ordinance of 1787, establishing public schools throughout the Northwest Territory; the Morrill Act of 1864, exchanging federal lands for state universities with expertise in engineering and agriculture; the late nineteenth-century Progressive movement, which emphasized professionally and efficiently run government; and the vast redistributive programs of the New Deal and Great Society administrations of Presidents Franklin Roosevelt and Lyndon

Johnson, respectively. Indeed, the New Federalism of the 1980s and 1990s, calling for a redefinition of federal government involvement in community and state affairs, is justified as a search for new, more responsive formulas that will better the lives of all Americans. Certainly the Republican party's "Contract with America" in the mid-1990s extended this quest. Regardless of presidential orientation, party politics, or prevailing ideology, Wilson's definition, coined nearly 100 years ago, remains today a valid statement of the appropriate and necessary role of government. Government's business, then, "is to establish and maintain every condition which will assist the people to a sound and wholesome and successful life."[50]

The "business" of bureaucracy is to serve as the primary trustee of resources and activities designed to maintain and enhance the human condition. The public service makes concrete the will of the people, as expressed through statutes, city ordinances, executive orders, and court decisions. Its external task, therefore, is to deliver public services, and in the process it forms a bridge of faith and trust between the citizenry and the Constitution.

The HIV/AIDS epidemic raises two fundamental concerns about the delivery of services and the resulting relationship between the public and its practitioners: what services will be provided, and who will deliver them? First, the quality or level of services delivered may diminish because government employs people within the HIV spectrum.[51] This seems to be a fear expressed by many public servants at all levels of government.

Exactly how many public servants are seropositive? As noted in Chapter 1, we cannot tell. With over 18 million employees, however, the government workforce is the largest in the United States.[52] Furthermore, we have every reason to assume that the epidemic affects people employed in the public sector in equal fashion and in the same proportions as it does those who work in the private sector. Given that as much as 1 percent of the American population might be HIV positive, as many as 180,000 government employees may currently fall within the HIV spectrum.

How does the employment of people in the HIV spectrum affect the quality of services delivered by government? As tables 4 and 5 indicate, workplace expenses associated with HIV/AIDS will continue to escalate as more employees become infected with the retrovirus and progress through the final stage of AIDS. As in the private sector, expenses borne by the public will include increased costs in health care benefits, sick leaves, group life insurance, reasonable accommodations, and recruitment and training of replacement personnel.

While the private sector can typically pass on such added expenses to the consumer, government cannot usually do so. HIV/AIDS thus necessitates difficult decisions about the allocation of scarce resources emanating from a limited, and in many cases shrinking, budget. Such is especially the case with municipal government; citizens of the 1990s appear less likely to approve increases in community tax levels, and the New Federalism has made local public servants more dependent upon local resources.

Table 6. Potential Impact of Employees with HIV/AIDS on Selected
Municipalities with Health Care Packages

Municipality	Approx. Size Workforce	HIV+ Projected No.	Estimated Cost[a]
Mt. Pleasant, MI	100	1	$ 136,000
Statesboro, GA	200	2	272,000
Las Cruces, NM	900	9	1,224,000
Bakersfield, CA	1,100	11	1,496,000
Cleveland, OH	8,000	80	10,880,000
Los Angeles, CA	25,000	250	34,000,000

[a] Costs estimated over a thirteen-year period. See table 5.

Source: Adapted from Jack P. DeSario, Sue R. Faerman, and James D. Slack, *Local Government Information and Training Needs in the 21st Century* (Westport, CT: Quorum Books), 35.

Assuming a 1 percent infection rate, the conservative estimated cost, ranging from $136,000 to $210,000 for each employee with HIV/AIDS, might well translate into financial hardship for local government. The estimate that 110,000 municipal and county employees have HIV/AIDS means a workplace cost of the retrovirus that will range from $15 billion to over $23 billion for all local governments in the United States.[53] Table 6 projects the added, and most likely unexpected, costs that selected municipalities will incur as a result of having employees with HIV/AIDS.

Many local governments will have trouble maintaining current levels of service in the face of the mounting cost of employing seropositive individuals. Citizens might someday have to forgo preferred programs, perhaps in the areas of parks and recreation, public safety, or tourism and economic development, so that scarce resources can be reallocated to such personnel line items as insurance and sick leave. Programs that are either cut or reduced may be viewed by the citizenry not as luxury items but rather as services required to sustain economic prosperity and the quality of life within the community. The HIV/AIDS epidemic therefore obligates local government officials to address community expectations about the level of services while meeting the legal and health care requirements of workforce members. This problem is growing in urgency, given the fact that the epidemic continues to penetrate the fabric of all communities and regions.

A second area of fundamental concern is the manner in which services are delivered. This concern reflects partly epidemiological evidence and partly the American culture. Fear has special ramifications for the workplace in the public sector.[54] The issue here is the absence of certainty about the spread of the retrovirus; the possibility exists that fluid-to-blood transmission can be accomplished through work-related contact with open sores or wounds.[55] One question will therefore have to be addressed: in what situations is it safe for the public servant to have direct contact with citizens and coworkers in the age of AIDS?

While there is genuine concern on both sides of the citizen–public servant re-lationship, little can be done about the HIV-positive citizen. One of the basic prem-ises of public administration, after all, is that services must be delivered in an equi-table fashion. But street-level bureaucrats—those who come into daily and direct personal contact with all types of citizens—are delivering services in a different way. They are taking special precautions in dealing with the public. For instance, police now use rubber gloves when confronting demonstrators who may include mem-bers of the AIDS Coalition to Unleash Power (ACT-UP), a militant group that in-cludes seropositive individuals and demands better and more timely governmental responses to the epidemic. Such public confrontations can lead to fluid-to-blood contact between law enforcement personnel and people with HIV/AIDS in the crowd.[56] In the resuscitation of individuals, too, emergency medical staff and fire-fighters now use a special apparatus that prevents direct mouth-to-mouth contact. Despite the latest epidemiological evidence about HIV/AIDS, many rescue per-sonnel refuse to perform direct mouth-to-mouth procedures because they are afraid of contracting the retrovirus through contact with blood in either saliva or vomit.

From the citizen's perspective, the HIV/AIDS epidemic is also raising ques-tions about *who* is delivering critical services. For the most part, the public seems rational about the employment of seropositive workers in areas such as street main-tenance and water departments or as administrators and employees at city hall. Some citizens may not like the fact that people with HIV/AIDS may work in the city's budget office, but their health is not threatened because their contact with these individuals is more limited. Practitioners in the HIV spectrum holding such positions are not really at issue.

Some citizens might object, however, if a seropositive firefighter, bleeding from falling debris, rescued an injured child from a burning building. Even in the absence of sound epidemiological evidence, some members of the community might ques-tion a seropositive lifeguard's administration of direct, mouth-to-mouth resuscita-tion to a drowning child at a public swimming pool.[57] In each scenario the child has a slim chance of survival without immediate assistance and intervention. The chances of contracting HIV/AIDS in these situations are also extremely slim, but they are not diminished by the fact that, in all likelihood, neither the firefighter nor the lifeguard is aware of being seropositive. Many people would probably prefer that government not permit individuals known to be within the HIV spectrum to hold positions in emergency-response occupations.

On the external side of bureaucracy, therefore, the HIV/AIDS epidemic raises concerns about future levels of services as well as about the appropriate manner in which services are delivered. These concerns bear directly on the relationship be-tween citizen and public servant and affect bureaucracy's role in maintaining the human condition. At the heart of the issue lie two questions: How safe is the public sector workplace? How healthy is the public sector workforce?

The Internal Side of Bureaucracy

Before we can answer questions about the nature of the public sector workplace and workforce, we must examine the internal side of bureaucracy. Both formal and informal policies, practices, and managerial attitudes define and direct basic human resource management activities, such as the employment and maintenance of the workforce, the assignment of individuals to positions within the workplace, appropriate patterns of interaction and communications, and appropriate procedures for separation and dismissal from the organization.

The HIV/AIDS epidemic raises four key questions about the internal dynamics of bureaucracy. First and most fundamental, how prepared is government to address workplace ramifications of the retrovirus? Second, what are appropriate ways to select and screen public employees in the age of AIDS? Third, does HIV/AIDS change the nature of confidentiality for public employees? Fourth, what are the appropriate kinds of contact between public servants in the HIV spectrum and citizens or other coworkers? These questions constitute the major themes addressed throughout the remainder of this book.

Government Preparedness

The question of government preparedness in dealing with HIV/AIDS in government's own workplace is a curious one. After all, bureaucracy does not really lack the requisite skills, knowledge, and training capacity to resolve the organizational dimensions of the HIV/AIDS crisis. Government has endured many natural disasters and public emergencies throughout history, and it has developed organizational strategies that are routinely applied to each new situation.[58] What seems to be absent here is the knowledge of how emergency management skills and techniques might be applied to address workplace ramifications of the HIV/AIDS epidemic.

The primary reason for such a lack of knowledge is that the HIV/AIDS epidemic presents a truly unique type of public emergency to the practitioner. On the surface, it would appear an easy task to manage the effects of this epidemic in the workplace. The retrovirus does not strike randomly in the same sense as other public disasters. In contrast to tornadoes and hurricanes, professionals can forecast and even chart the course of HIV/AIDS well in advance of its entry into specific workforces. The path of HIV/AIDS, for instance, is known to affect workforces in larger cities initially and then to penetrate the fabric of smaller communities. We can track its progress from coastal areas in the mid-1980s into the nation's heartland in the mid-1990s and later. We should therefore be able to predict with a higher degree of confidence (as we cannot with natural and technological emergencies) that the retrovirus will soon infect public and private workforces (if it has not done so already) in such disparate and remote communities as Athens, Ohio, and Athens, Georgia.

Yet the reality of the situation makes it much harder to manage such a public emergency. For instance, it is extremely difficult to tell exactly when the HIV/AIDS disaster will hit the workplace. Tornadoes and hurricanes leave immediate indicators of death and destruction, as do fires in theaters, restaurants, or other public facilities. Such evidence of natural disasters makes possible a relatively precise record and timetable of the emergency. Even with technological emergencies, the start of the disaster can be pinpointed with relatively little difficulty; toxic leaks and chemical spills are easily detected. Because people know when these crises occur, furthermore, experts also know when to set into motion a host of response-oriented activities. Such knowledge ultimately helps public administration apply resources and skills to the situation.

Unfortunately the same is not true of HIV/AIDS. Unless HIV antibody blood testing has been administered, or symptoms of AIDS are manifest, individuals may not even know that they are in the HIV spectrum. Furthermore, as a result of the social stigma attached to the epidemic, the public continues to label related illnesses in ways intended to dissociate the person's impending death from HIV/ AIDS. When someone dies from a tornado or a chemical disaster, the information is reported in front-page newspaper stories as well as in obituaries. Far too frequently, however, readers must still speculate as to whether or not an individual died of HIV/AIDS.

While it is easier to forecast public emergencies in the case of HIV/AIDS than with other disasters, confirming its existence can be a more prolonged, politically sensitive, and costly process. Our inability to verify the presence of HIV/AIDS reinforces the illusion that there is no emergency. Because public administrators cannot pinpoint the disease's time of arrival in the workforce, the implementation of responses in the workplace yields to politically and culturally based delays that would not be factors in the event of other types of natural and technological crises.

Preparation for the workplace ramifications of HIV/AIDS, and management of them, requires planning. Even if it is difficult to verify that the retrovirus is on hand in the public sector workforce, we can still anticipate its arrival and begin to develop strategies. We might start by asking whether government has established formal plans and guidelines for coping with the retrovirus in its workforce. An HIV/AIDS plan comprises: (1) a statement supporting the civil rights of all employees who are in the HIV spectrum, (2) a set of procedures that should be followed in dealing with seropositive employees, (3) a set of services available to seropositive employees, and (4) a plan to train and retrain supervisors on a systematic basis. If government has not adopted an official HIV/AIDS plan, then has it developed other strategies to address the workplace ramifications of HIV/ AIDS?

Selection and Screening

The second issue deals with the selection and screening of public employees. Here government must search for a legal and equitable formula to protect the service delivery needs of the community and the civil rights of the employee with HIV/AIDS. Major questions include: under what conditions must local government hire and retain job applicants and employees in the HIV spectrum? What are the legal parameters in determining whether employees and job applicants can be tested for HIV/AIDS? Should HIV antibody blood testing be mandatory for all workers? Should employers test only certain categories of workers, say job applicants or those who may find themselves in fluid-to-blood contact with coworkers or citizens?[59] How accurate are test results? What does a positive test result actually tell management about a specific employee?

Confidentiality

The issue of screening leads to the third concern affecting the internal dynamics of bureaucracy. There must be a balance between the worker's right to maintain confidentiality in all health-related matters and the twofold responsibility of professional public management: (1) to ensure the citizen's right to be informed about issues that may affect government's ability to deliver services and (2) to provide necessary information within the organization to allow for its appropriate and effective functioning.

Typically Americans believe that the public has a right to know what goes on at city hall. The democratic tradition presupposes that citizens have sufficient information to make rational decisions about every aspect of government, including the allocation of tax-base resources. Can a citizen vote intelligently on requests for tax increases for preferred programs, such as a new municipal sport stadium or additional schools, if she does not possess actual or projected costs of other items that may or may not be affected by the number of persons in the HIV spectrum employed by government? In order to make intelligent decisions, how much information about HIV/AIDS in the workplace must a citizen have? Is it necessary to know which departments employ people in the HIV spectrum, or will the total number employed throughout the municipal organization suffice? Does a citizen have a right to know the names of public servants in the HIV spectrum? If HIV antibody testing is conducted in the workplace, to what degree should the results remain confidential? In what situations, and in what form, should test results be disclosed to the public?

The question of confidentiality is also germane to the operation of the workplace. On the one hand, people's medical records are presumed to be confidential as long as their health condition does not endanger the health of those around them. Yet a balance must be struck between the employee's right to privacy and confidentiality and the organization's need to respond to the workplace ramifications of the retrovirus. Who within the organization needs to know that a particular employee has HIV/AIDS? Furthermore, if government is to be prepared to deal with the HIV/AIDS epidemic in its own workplace, does it not need to collect, aggregate, and analyze data on the well-being of its employees?

Contact with Citizens and Coworkers

The final concern about the internal side of bureaucracy focuses on the nature of contact between the worker with HIV/AIDS and others. The stakes are not simply epidemiological but also political. Here cultural factors may have their greatest bearing on behavior. The questions confronting government include the following: is it acceptable for the seropositive worker to have direct contact with members of the public at large, especially in situations that might result in fluid-to-blood contact? Is it acceptable to permit the worker to have direct contact with special groups, such as children? Municipal government officials must calculate the amount of actual and perceived risk they are prepared to take in light of the complex blend of scientific, political, and cultural issues.

Summary

The four concerns outlined above will be answered by epidemiological findings as well as by the boundaries developed in legislation, court decisions, and city ordinances. Within the confines of these parameters, however, the nation's political culture and social values will certainly play a role. Standard operating procedures can be influenced by the discretionary authority exercised by individual managers and administrators, all of whom embody American values. According to the eminent scholar Frederick C. Mosher, "The great bulk of decisions and actions taken by governments are determined or heavily influenced by administrative officials, most of whom are appointed, not elected."[60] We are also reminded by Frank J. Thompson of the political importance of the personnel function to most public managers. They tend to "live with the politics of jobs day in and day out, aware that their success in other policy arenas often depends on their ability to cope with personnel issues."[61] Much sooner than the public at large, practitioners will be aware of the drain on resources that is caused by the HIV/AIDS epidemic. The survival and future well-being of key units and programs within their organizations may very well be determined by the extent to which HIV/AIDS is present in members of their staffs.

The point here is that chief administrative officers and other supervisors in the chain of command can often help delineate the boundaries of discretion and responsibility. They can determine what practices and decision rules are acceptable and unacceptable. From this perspective, James M. Kouzes and Barry Z. Posner correctly note that organizational leadership constitutes "an active, not a passive process."[62] In the case of workplace ramifications of HIV/AIDS, the process of leadership is certainly not neutral. By either acting or not acting, expressing one's values or remaining silent on the key issues outlined above, managers and supervisors have an enormous opportunity to influence the tone of the organization in managing the HIV/AIDS epidemic.

Cultural factors help define the nature of governmental responses to the retrovirus in general as well as to the many workplace ramifications of the epidemic. I have argued that HIV/AIDS is creating a special crisis in the public service. The bureaucracy represents the employer of the largest number of people in this country and, unlike the private sector, has only rather limited means of adjusting budgets to cover new and unexpected costs. This statement is particularly true for local governments, whose employees comprise more than 60 percent of the total public service workforce.

From the perspective of the citizen, the consequences of the epidemic are becoming increasingly visible on the external side of bureaucracy. HIV/AIDS affects not only the level and quality of public services but also the manner in which those services are delivered. At the heart of the crisis, however, lie key decisions that are made about the internal workings of bureaucracy, issues pertaining to the nature of personnel as well as to the dynamics of the workplace environment. By addressing these internal concerns arising from the HIV/AIDS epidemic, government may better prepare itself to carry out its fundamental mission of improving the human condition through service delivery.

3

HIV/AIDS and the Law

WHILE MOST STATES and many municipalities have enacted legislation to protect the rights of the seropositive individual, this chapter focuses on protections provided by the federal government.[1] Federal legislation is important, after all, because it cannot be contravened by state laws or local ordinances. Organizations, whether in Boston or Bakersfield, must therefore comply with the rights protected by federal law as well as by the U.S. Constitution.

FEDERAL LEGISLATION

Two pieces of federal legislation are designed to protect the rights of job applicants and employees in the HIV spectrum as well as the rights of clients and citizens with HIV/AIDS who receive services from public agencies. These laws are the Rehabilitation Act and the Americans with Disabilities Act.[2] Organizations covered by either act are prohibited from discriminating against otherwise qualified persons with HIV/AIDS, including those who have just tested positive for the retrovirus and those who have contracted full-blown AIDS.[3] Management cannot discriminate in the design or application of recruitment, selection, promotion, retention, retirement, and termination policies and practices. Otherwise qualified disabled individuals cannot be denied access to various job-related and career advancement opportunities, such as training programs and professional development seminars. Otherwise qualified clients and citizens with HIV/AIDS, furthermore, cannot be denied access to, or benefits from, public services offered by either public or private entities covered under either act.

Differences Between the Rehab Act and the ADA

Both pieces of legislation are similar in terms of protections offered, but there are at least five important differences between the Rehab Act and the ADA.[4] First, there are differences in decision rules concerning the organizations that are covered under the acts. The Rehab Act, like many other regulatory policies, links coverage to the federal payroll and the intergovernmental funding system.[5] Those who qualify for protection are: (1) federal workers and individuals in federal programs, (2) employees of companies and agencies that receive federal government contracts in excess of $2,500, and (3) employees of agencies that receive funds and assistance from the federal government. As recipients of federal funding, most municipal governments are covered under the Rehab Act.[6]

The ADA, on the other hand, has much broader coverage because it is not tied to federal funding.[7] It covers organizations engaged in an "industry affecting commerce" and with "15 or more employees for each working day in each of 20 or more calendar weeks in the current or preceding calendar year."[8] Because Congress takes a very eclectic view of the phrase "industry affecting commerce," most municipal governments are covered by the ADA as well as by the Rehab Act.

The second difference between the Rehab Act and the ADA concerns their respective policy missions.[9] The Rehab Act requires organizations to be "disability-conscious." Organizations covered by it must take affirmative action in the hiring and promotion processes and must report annually to the Equal Employment Opportunity Commission on the success of their affirmative action efforts.[10] The ADA, however, requires covered organizations to be "disability-blind." Its sole purpose is to eliminate discrimination against individuals with disabilities, and it includes no affirmative action component.[11] For most municipalities, as well as other organizations covered by both acts, the need to be simultaneously "disability-conscious" and "disability-blind" can lead to confusion and frustration as managers engage in the various personnel processes.

The third distinction between the two pieces of federal legislation has to do with enforcement mechanisms. While due process under both laws can take more than one year, seeking remedy under the Rehab Act involves a much more complex process. Grievances against the federal government as employer are handled by the EEOC, while claims against private companies are channeled through the Office of Federal Contract Compliance Programs.[12] The enforcement responsibilities for claims against organizations that receive federal monies and programs, including municipal governments, rest with the funding source (department or agency) within the federal government, and efforts are coordinated by the U.S. Justice Department.[13] In contrast, the process of seeking remedy under the ADA is quite straightforward. The ADA requires that all claims against employers be handled through the EEOC.[14]

The fourth difference between the two acts pertains to architectural requirements for barrier removal. The Rehab Act uses stricter requirements and employs the term "must accommodate" in removing all barriers that deny disabled individuals access to jobs and services.[15] The ADA, on the other hand, is somewhat more lenient and uses the term "readily achievable" in relationship to the removal of barriers. "Readily achievable" means that an architectural task is "easily accomplishable and able to be carried out without much difficulty or expense."[16]

Differences in the language on barrier removal can affect municipal government. For instance, assume that the City of Bakersfield, California, occupies a building that does not have wheelchair-accessible stalls in the rest rooms. (Perhaps the building is old and the rest rooms are too small for such stalls.) If the building houses a program that receives federal funding, it is covered under the Rehab Act. Accordingly, the city is required to remove the architectural barriers to the building and to expand the rest rooms to make the necessary modifications.

If the same municipal building houses no programs receiving federal funding, it is most likely covered under the ADA. It might not have to make structural adjustments to the existing building if it cannot do so in a "readily achievable" manner.[17] The ADA, however, will still require the city to devise less expensive ways to make the rest rooms more accessible to disabled individuals, perhaps by constructing a new one out of prefabricated material in a central part of the building.

The final difference between the two acts relates to the terms "handicap" and "disability." The term "handicap" is used throughout the Rehab Act, while the term "disability" is used with the ADA. While on the surface the difference may seem semantic, the two words are important legal keys to the efficient use of either piece of legislation. Let's assume that an employee or job applicant with HIV/AIDS believes himself to be the victim of workplace discrimination in a municipal department that receives federal funding. To request a remedy under the Rehab Act, he must file a claim with the appropriate federal funding agency and designate himself a "handicapped" person. This procedure is especially important if he wishes to file charges under the affirmative action sections of the act. On the other hand, if the job applicant or employee with HIV/AIDS believes she is the victim of workplace discrimination in a municipality that receives no federal funding or in a department that receives no such funding, to request a remedy through the ADA she must designate herself a "disabled" person.[18]

Similarities Between the Rehab Act and the ADA

Except for the points noted above, the Rehab Act and the ADA are identical pieces of legislation. They have the same purpose of protecting the workplace rights of people with disabilities or handicaps, including persons within the HIV spectrum, as well as the same definition of "disability/handicap."[19] The requirements of notification and documentation are the same for job applicants and employees under both pieces of legislation, as are the responsibilities of management.

According to both pieces of legislation, a handicapped or disabled person is someone with:

1. a physical or mental impairment that substantially limits one or more of the major life activities of such individual;
2. a record of such an impairment; or
3. being regarded as having such an impairment.[20]

Because the Rehab Act was enacted prior to the HIV/AIDS epidemic, neither the specific language of the law nor the legislative intent addresses the pertinent ramifications of the retrovirus. Throughout the 1980s, however, a series of administrative rulings and court cases reaffirmed the rights of people with HIV/AIDS under this act. In an administrative law action, *Doe v. Charlotte Memorial Hospital,* the Office of Civil Rights of the U.S. Department of Health and Human Services reasoned that the hospital could not prevent a nurse who had been diagnosed with HIV/AIDS from working when evidence was shown that she could not infect others.[21] In *Arline,* a case involving a schoolteacher who had contracted tuberculosis, the Supreme Court stated that simply having a contagious disease is not sufficient reason by itself to deny a person access to employment if evidence suggests that the disease would not be spread when precautions were taken in the workplace.[22] The high court concluded, therefore, that people in such situations were protected under the Rehab Act.

In *Thomas,* a case that dealt with a child in the HIV spectrum with a habit of biting, a federal court determined that a person with HIV/AIDS was "handicapped" within the meaning of the Rehab Act.[23] The court ruled that even though Ryan Thomas had HIV/AIDS, he could attend kindergarten because he was "otherwise qualified" to do so. According to the court:

> The overwhelming weight of medical evidence is that the AIDS virus is not transmitted by human bites, even bites that break the skin. Based upon the abundant medical and scientific evidence before the Court, Ryan poses no risk of harm to his classmates and teachers. Any theoretical risk of transmission of the AIDS virus by Ryan in connection with his attendance in regular kindergarten class is so remote that it cannot form the basis for any exclusionary action by the School District.[24]

The *Chalk* decision dealt with a teacher within the HIV spectrum who had direct contact with students. A school district in California was successful in persuading a lower court to prevent Vincent L. Chalk from returning to the classroom because he had HIV/AIDS.[25] The Ninth District Court of Appeals, however, ruled that no evidence existed to suggest that casual, *work-related* behavior and contact would cause the transmission of HIV/AIDS. Furthermore, the court ruled that Vincent Chalk "was not required to disprove every theoretical possibility of harm" and that the "possibility that [his] return to the classroom would produce fear and apprehension in parents and students was not grounds" for denying him access to the workplace.

The decision in the *Leckelt* case reaffirmed the court's position against discrimination on the basis of a "perceived disability" and therefore underscored the right of protection under the third ("regarded as having") definition of handicap for asymptomatic seropositive people.[26] Here a hospital employee's roommate contracted HIV/AIDS and was admitted into the same hospital. The hospital administrator insisted that the plaintiff take an HIV antibody blood test and have the test results reported to the hospital. The plaintiff refused and was subsequently terminated. While the court ruled in favor of the hospital, it was emphatic in noting that it did so only because the discharged nurse had failed to establish that the hospital had perceived him as being seropositive.

The legislative history of the ADA makes it clear that Congress intended to incorporate these judicial rulings in the law and meant to include people within the HIV spectrum under the act.[27] The retrovirus and its resultant illnesses constitute physical and mental impairments that affect the major life activities as outlined by Congress: walking, seeing, hearing, speaking, breathing, learning, working, performing manual tasks, and caring for oneself.[28] HIV/AIDS also passes the threefold test, established by the EEOC, to determine whether or not specific impairments *substantially limit* these life activities:

1. What is the nature and severity of the impairment?
2. What is the impairment's duration?
3. What is the permanent and long-term impact of the impairment?[29]

Given the incumbent and interpretive language associated with both pieces of legislation, and our knowledge of the various stages of the retrovirus, it is clear that job applicants and employees in the HIV spectrum can claim protection under each of the three definitions of "disability."[30] Someone with either persistent generalized lymphadenopathy or full-blown AIDS qualifies as a disabled worker under the first definition (having an actual physical or mental impairment). An individual with full-blown AIDS, however, will sometimes temporarily recover from one or a combination of the opportunistic diseases or AIDS-related cancers. As an example, a person might contract *Pneumocystis carinii* pneumonia or pulmonary cytomegalovirus—both common opportunistic infections from which many PLWAs recover only to succumb to them once again at a later date. Or a person might have the malignancy Kaposi's sarcoma (KS), but it may fall into a state of remission. In all such situations, she or he qualifies under the second definition (having a record of a physical or mental impairment).

In addition, seroconverted persons are protected under the third definition (they are regarded as having a physical or mental impairment).[31] Protection here can extend to a wide variety of persons within the HIV spectrum, ranging from those who are in the asymptomatic stage to people still asymptomatic but with CD_4 T-cell counts below 200 (full-blown AIDS). These people are still regarded as "disabled" under the ADA, and "handicapped" under the Rehab Act, because of the 100 percent fatality rate of HIV infection. Given that perhaps millions of people in the United States are unknowingly HIV positive and asymptomatic, this category of disability will become the one most commonly used in the future.

RESPONSIBILITIES OF THE JOB APPLICANT AND EMPLOYEE

The responsibilities of the seropositive job applicant and employee are few but critically important for protection from workplace discrimination. In essence, both the Rehab Act and the ADA require a process of self-empowerment. Workplace protection demands that the PLWA provide management with official notification and documentation establishing that she has either the retrovirus or related illnesses.[32] The person must also provide management with notification and documentation of specific impairments when seeking specific workplace assistance.

It is important to note that management is not obligated to protect the rights of disabled individuals, including those within the HIV spectrum, when it does not know of the existence of specific impairments.[33] When notification and documentation do not occur, some managers might conceivably choose to engage in activities designed to get rid of the employee who is "suspected" of having HIV/AIDS. Equally important, persons with HIV/AIDS must submit self-identifying proof of seropositivity, such as a nonanonymous HIV antibody blood test result or a physician's report saying that they have the retrovirus, as part of the documentation process in order to gain full protection from workplace discrimination. An anonymous test result cannot be used because it does not directly and officially link a person with HIV/AIDS.

MANAGEMENT'S RESPONSIBILITIES

Management's responsibilities are extensive under both the Rehab Act and the ADA. They involve: (1) determining the essential functions of each job assignment, (2) using appropriate screening devices, (3) providing reasonable accommodations, (4) understanding and knowing when to claim undue hardship, (5) dealing with the issue of confidentiality, and (6) dealing with the issue of contact with employees with HIV/AIDS.

Essential Functions of the Job

According to both acts, a qualified individual with a disability is someone who "with or without reasonable accommodation, can perform the essential functions of the employment position that such individual holds or desires."[34] In order to know whether a person with HIV/AIDS is otherwise qualified for a position—that is, whether one can do the job with or without reasonable accommodation—management must first identify the essential functions of the job.[35] These are the primary and central job tasks of the position. EEOC requires that three factors be taken into consideration in determining whether or not a specific job task is actually an essential function of the position: (1) the particular task must be so central that it is the reason why the position was created, (2) the particular task must be so specialized that only a minimum number of employees can perform its task, and (3) the particular task in question must be so technical that the person holding the job was recruited specifically to perform it.[36]

It is management's responsibility to differentiate between the essential functions and the marginal ones in each position within the organization. Once the essential functions are determined, job descriptions should be restructured to reflect the nature and importance of these tasks. In order to determine whether a job applicant with HIV/AIDS is otherwise qualified, essential functions of the job in question should be listed in all job advertisements and should be the focal point of the job interview. For a job description that distinguishes between essential and marginal functions, see Appendix D.

Screening of Job Applicants with HIV/AIDS

As noted above, both the Rehab Act and the ADA protect seropositive job applicants as well as employees.[37] Using language identical to that found in the Rehab Act, the ADA states that employers cannot deny access to job opportunities by "using qualification standards, employment tests or other selection criteria that screen out or tend to screen out an individual with a disability or class of individuals with disabilities."[38]

Management can use screening devices in the hiring process only when such devices meet two conditions.[39] First, the screening device must be job related. That is, it must test directly and solely the essential functions of the position. For instance, it would clearly be acceptable to require an applicant for a clerical position to demonstrate word-processing skills. Eliminating a person from the pool of clerical job applicants on the basis of KS lesions on his or her face, however, would not meet the job-related standard, nor in most cases would requiring the applicant for a clerical position to drive a car for the purpose of running errands marginal to the job's function.[40]

Second, the screening device must be "consistent with business necessity" and must take into consideration the nature of the entity.[41] For instance, the use of X-rays as a screening device to determine the possibility of future injury would probably be deemed not consistent with business necessity for a driver of a municipal sanitation truck.[42] The use of X-rays as a screening device might, however, be regarded as consistent with business necessity if the business in question was a franchise in the National Football League and the job advertisement was for a quarterback. Similarly, it might not be consistent with business necessity to require a hearing test for a position in the city's personnel or budget office because of the nature of job tasks in these offices.[43] It would be consistent with business necessity to require a driver's license for the position of municipal bus driver, however, and it would also address the job-relatedness criteria.[44]

Interview Questions

Interview questions constitute a common screening device, and much of the implicit discrimination against persons with HIV/AIDS takes place during the interviews.[45] The following are some of the questions and comments that are inappropriate for job interviews:

1. Do you have HIV?
2. Please list any AIDS-related conditions that you have had in the past three years.
3. Have you ever been hospitalized as a result of having HIV/AIDS?
4. Have you ever been treated by a psychiatrist or psychologist for HIV/AIDS?
5. Have you ever been treated for any HIV/AIDS-related mental condition?
6. Is there any HIV/AIDS-related health problem that might keep you from performing the job for which you are applying?
7. Are you taking any antiviral drugs or protease inhibitors?
8. Have you ever filed for workers' compensation insurance?[46]

Medical Examinations

Another common screening device in the hiring process is medical or physical examinations. The Rehab Act and the ADA prohibit the use of such examinations as a preemployment screening device except when such tests are deemed job related and consistent with business necessity.[47] At the municipal government level, such preemployment examinations tend to constitute a legal screening device for selected positions within the police and fire departments as well as for entrance into the police academy.[48] Management may require a medical examination after making an offer to a job applicant and may make the offer of employment conditional upon acceptable results from the medical examination if:

1. all entering employees are subjected to such an examination regardless of disability;
2. information obtained regarding the medical condition or history of the applicant is collected and maintained on separate forms and in separate medical files and is treated as a confidential medical record;
3. the results of such examination are used only in accordance with this title.[49]

In what situations can management withdraw the job offer as a result of the postoffer, preemployment physical examination? As with most issues dealing with the Rehab Act and the ADA, the question will be answered on a case-by-case basis. Below is one example from EEOC involving the withdrawal of the job offer on the basis of the findings of the postoffer, preemployment medical examination.

[A]n employer makes a conditional offer of employment to an applicant, and it is an essential function of the job that the incumbent be available to work every day for the next three months. An employment entrance examination then reveals that the applicant has a disabling impairment that, according to reasonable medical judgment that relies on the most current medical knowledge, will require treatment that will render the applicant unable to work for a portion of the three month period. Under these circumstances, the employer would be able to withdraw the employment offer.[50]

HIV Testing

Can employers screen job applicants by using an HIV antibody blood test as part of a postoffer, preemployment medical examination?[51] In certain situations managers can use HIV tests for such purposes. It is important for managers to understand what is involved in the testing procedure, however, and what the test results actually mean. An explanation of these factors appears in Appendix B.

HIV antibody testing produces anxiety not only because of potential medical results but also because of the potential political uses of test results.[52] When HIV antibody testing is used as a screening device in the workplace, it becomes mandatory for those seeking employment and career opportunities. Job applicants or employees have little choice but to take the test or jeopardize their future with the organization.

Since the beginning of the epidemic, various public sector employers have embraced mandatory HIV antibody testing. These efforts tend to fail when they are too broadly construed and violate guarantees of privacy in the U.S. Constitution. Privacy, in the form of protection from searches and seizures, is the central concern of the Fourth Amendment, which reads in part: "The right of the people to be secure in their persons, houses, papers, and effects, against unreasonable searches and seizures, shall not be violated."

The courts have established that the drawing of blood, as well as other bodily fluids, is a form of search.[53] Mandatory HIV antibody testing in the workplace must balance the individual's right to privacy with the government's interest in knowing who has been exposed to the virus.

The federal government has implemented a series of mandatory HIV screening programs since the mid-1980s.[54] Department of Defense testing began on a selective basis in 1985. Currently, HIV testing is mandatory for all new military recruits, all cadets in the service academies, and all individuals on active duty. Civilian employees of the Department of Defense are exempt. The reasons for testing are foreign governments' concern that HIV-infected GIs might introduce the disease in their countries and the need to keep a healthy workforce in the "combat workplace" where crisis may dictate the sharing of a blood supply.

HIV antibody testing is mandatory for all members of the Foreign Service. The requirement reflects a belief that foreign governments might place seropositive employees in compromising positions and, as with combat situations in the military, that embassy staff might need to depend on their own blood supply in times of crisis.[55]

In the Job Corps (Department of Labor), HIV antibody testing is mandatory for all applicants and trainers. The rationale for testing is the need to halt the spread of HIV. Testing is also mandatory for all prisoners in federal penitentiaries and for all new immigrants to the United States; by testing, authorities hope to gain knowledge that will help keep the disease from spreading.

Most states have established mandatory HIV antibody testing procedures for inmates in correctional facilities. County and municipal judges also commonly order mandatory HIV antibody testing, especially in cases involving rape or other sexual offenses. The courts have also upheld the right of municipalities to institute mandatory HIV testing programs for specific groups, especially firefighters, paramedics, and police officers.[56] It is important to underscore that, although the courts have condoned mandatory HIV antibody testing in certain situations, they have never permitted the results of screening, or knowledge of a person's HIV status, to be used to discriminate against employees who, with or without reasonable accommodation, can perform the essential functions of the job.[57]

In general, it is legal to employ an HIV antibody blood test as a screening device within the guidelines set forth by the Rehab Act and the ADA. The employer must show that the screening procedure is (1) narrowly focused, (2) job related, (3) consistent with business necessity, and (4) administered to all employees in a particular classification or throughout the entire organization. As Walter J. Jones and James A. Johnson point out, however, "the legal burden of proof will almost always be on the organization to show specifically why job requirements mandate an inquiry into the health status of the employee or applicant."[58]

Reasonable Accommodation

Under both the Rehab Act and the ADA, management is required to provide reasonable accommodation to disabled job applicants and employees, including people with HIV/AIDS, who request assistance in performing the essential functions of their jobs.[59] Failure to provide reasonable accommodation can not only lead to claims of employment discrimination, it can also result in litigation claiming both negligent and intentional infliction of emotional distress.[60] But what is reasonable accommodation? Here again, the answer will be determined on a case-by-case basis.[61] Suggestions and guidelines for defining reasonable accommodations in specific settings are available from several sources. The Job Accommodation Network, for instance, assists individual employers in this effort, as do several university-based outreach units across the country.[62]

The EEOC and Congress offer the following decision rules:

1. Reasonable accommodations do not have to be the "best" or the "most expensive," but they do need to be "sufficient" for performing the essential functions of the job.
2. Management must cover the cost of the reasonable accommodations when such accommodations are used exclusively at the workplace.
3. Management must pay a proportion of the cost of reasonable accommoda-

tions, such as wheel chairs or computer equipment in homes, that are used during working hours.

4. Management is not responsible for providing reasonable accommodations for disabilities about which it has not received official notification and documentation.

5. Management cannot provide reasonable accommodations unless they are specifically requested by the job applicant or employee.[63]

Gary S. Marx and Gary G. Goldberger suggest using the following four-step approach in developing reasonable and effective accommodations:

1. *Determine the fundamental job tasks.* Analyzing the fundamental job tasks means simply making a list of each task that will need to be performed by the employee.

2. *Determine the individual's abilities.* The applicant should be analyzed on an individual basis to determine his abilities and limitations, such as his ability to lip-read or hear the telephone ring.

3. *Determine conflicts between fundamental job tasks and the individual's abilities.* The results of the first and second steps should be compared in order to determine whether any incompatibilities exist.

4. *Determine and evaluate solutions to those conflicts.* If any conflicts are found, accommodations (i.e., solutions) should be considered and made.[64]

Using language similar to that in the Rehab Act, the ADA indicates that reasonable accommodations may include two types of activities. First, *general* changes in the organization might be made to allow for greater access to and within the workplace. Second, *specific* changes in the job in question—its nature or the way it is conducted—might be made to enhance the disabled person's ability to perform the essential task functions. According to the ADA, reasonable accommodations may consist of:

1. making existing facilities used by employees readily accessible to and usable by individuals with disabilities; and

2. job restructuring, part-time or modified work schedules, reassignment to a vacant position, acquisition or modification of equipment or devices, appropriate adjustment or modifications of examinations, training materials or policies, the provision of qualified readers or interpreters, and other similar accommodations for individuals with disabilities.[65]

Examples of general changes, which might be considered as reasonable accommodations, include the installation of wheelchair ramps inside and outside buildings, placing braille signs and instructions in every elevator, and lowering the level of water fountains so that they may be used by people in wheelchairs. Examples of specific changes might include adapting an individual's work station computer to respond to voice commands, providing a computer modem and allowing the person to work at home, and awarding a person extra sick days if needed.

While it may be difficult for workplace managers and supervisors to define and apply the general concept of reasonable accommodation to specific situations involving different types of disabilities, HIV by its nature complicates the process. Because AIDS is a fatal disease, it is not unusual for the initial diagnosis of HIV to cast the person into a state of shock for a period lasting from several months to well over a year. Someone testing positive for HIV can do little but remain as healthy as possible, minimize levels of stress, search for and secure the services of a physician who is knowledgeable about HIV/AIDS and with whom a treatment strategy can be devised, hope that the success of protease inhibitors continues and their availability increases, and pray that a cure is discovered before he or she dies.

HIV-positive job applicants and employees require reasonable accommodations—even in the absence of clinical symptoms—because of the fundamentally life-taking nature of the retrovirus. Under the Rehab Act and the ADA, seropositive asymptomatic individuals have as much right as other disabled Americans to workplace-related assistance that will enable them to perform the essential functions of the job. Reasonable accommodations will keep them healthier longer and will make them less costly and more productive to the organization.

The many illnesses related to full-blown AIDS add to the complications in providing reasonable accommodations. As the immune system deteriorates, opportunistic diseases begin to attack the body sequentially and in combination. Someone with fungal infections, such as *Candida albicans* (thrush) or toxoplasmosis, might require different kinds of reasonable accommodations from someone with bacterial infections like *Mycobacterium avium* complex (MAC) or tuberculosis. Someone with viral infections, such as CMV or *Herpes Zoster* (shingles), might require yet another type of reasonable accommodation.[66] People taking one or a combination of antiviral drugs also tend to experience many side effects that might also require reasonable accommodations.[67] The strict regimen accompanying the use of protease inhibitors, for instance taking the drugs with a fatty meal at precise times throughout the day and night, will certainly require some workplace modifications. As Chapter 1 suggests, learning that one's CD_4 T-cell count has dropped dramatically might require additional, temporary accommodations similar to those needed immediately after the initial diagnosis of either HIV or full-blown AIDS. Each illness and situation—indeed, each individual at each stage of the disease—requires careful analysis to determine appropriate and effective reasonable accommodations.

Undue Hardship

To what extent must management provide reasonable accommodations to otherwise qualified job applicants and employees with HIV/AIDS? Stated another way, how "reasonable" must reasonable be? According to *Alexander v. Choate*, a balanced approach must be taken in establishing reasonable accommodations. The court determined that the particular strategy selected by the employer to achieve reasonable accommodation must pursue the objectives of the Rehab Act while remaining manageable in terms of the organization's capabilities.[68]

While *Alexander v. Choate* was decided prior to enactment of the ADA, its logic also appears in that act. Management does not have to provide a specific accommodation that causes the organization to incur a "significant difficulty or expense."[69] Using language similar to that in the Rehab Act, the ADA provides that the following factors must be taken into consideration when management determines whether a request for a specific accommodation imposes an undue hardship on the organization:

1. the nature and cost of the accommodation needed;
2. the overall financial resources of the facility or facilities involved in the provision of the reasonable accommodation; the number of persons employed at such facility; the effect on expenses and resources, or the impact otherwise of such accommodation upon the operation of the facility;
3. the overall financial resources of the covered entity; the overall size of the business of a covered entity with respect to the number of its employees; the number, type, and location of its facilities; and
4. the type of operation or operations of the covered entity, including the composition, structure, and functions of the work force of such entity; the geographic separateness, administrative, or fiscal relationship of the facility or facilities in question to the covered entity.[70]

EEOC *Interpretive Guidelines* do not require that undue hardship claims be based only on financial difficulties, although such issues lie at the heart of management's concerns and fears. Management also has a right to claim that a request for a specific accommodation is unduly disruptive to the workplace.[71] EEOC gives the following example:

> [A]n individual with a disabling visual impairment that makes it extremely difficult to see in dim lighting applies for a position as a waiter in a nightclub and requests that the club be brightly lit as a reasonable accommodation. Although the individual may be able to perform the job in bright lighting, the nightclub will probably be able to demonstrate that particular accommodation, though inexpensive, would be an undue hardship if the bright light would destroy the ambience of the nightclub and/or make it difficult for the customers to see the stage show.[72]

Organizations cannot claim, however, that employing people with disabilities, including individuals with HIV/AIDS, disrupts the workplace unduly. Nor can management argue that requests for reasonable accommodation are unduly disruptive because such requests might adversely impact the morale of coworkers or, in the case of municipalities, because they might elicit disapproval from citizens and members of city council. In essence, both the Rehab Act and the ADA disallow prejudices and unfounded fears as the basis for claims of undue hardship.[73]

In addition, an employer cannot deny employment opportunities to a disabled job applicant or employee simply because of current or future costs. The courts were clear on this issue before the passage of the ADA. In *Chrysler v. DILHR,* for instance, a person with leukemia was denied employment because the employer feared high absenteeism and an increase in copayments for health care benefits.[74] In *Western Weighing Bureau v. DILHR,* a job applicant was denied employment because he had a weak lower back and the company worried that he would get hurt on the job and would subsequently file for workers' compensation.[75] Similarly, in *Sterling Transit Co. v. FEPC*[76] and *E. E. Black Limited v. Marshall,* persons were denied employment because of back problems.[77] In *McDermott v. Xerox,* a handicapped person was refused a job from fear that life insurance premiums would eventually rise. In each of these cases, the courts ruled that it is unlawful to discriminate against the disabled individual and that insufficient action had been taken to effect the reasonable accommodation intent of federal and state legislation.[78]

In the case of HIV/AIDS, courts have also generally ruled in favor of the HIV employee.[79] For instance, Hyatt Legal Services was forced to pay over $150,000 in damages to an individual who was fired after he informed the company that he was HIV infected. In *Cain v. Joel Hyatt,* the U.S. district court ruled that "an employer's conclusion that a given person will be physically unable to satisfy job requirements in the long-run almost always will rest on inherently speculative grounds."[80] In effect, the court reasoned that the company did not comply with its duty of accommodation.

What constitutes an undue hardship for a municipal government as it confronts HIV/AIDS in the workplace? Since municipalities will certainly differ in the capacity to make reasonable accommodations, they will also vary in the ability to afford certain accommodations. Once again, the claim of undue hardship will be made on a case-by-case basis.

The law and EEOC *Interpretive Guidelines,* however, do suggest some reliable guidelines. Despite the fact that they have more employees, managers in city governments with larger overall operating budgets will most likely have to pursue reasonable accommodations farther before claiming undue hardship than will their counterparts in smaller settings with smaller revenue bases. In all likelihood, however, the presence of only one person with HIV/AIDS in the workforce of a small rural municipality does not give that organization carte blanche in claiming undue hardship. Regardless of the size of the budget or workforce, municipal governments will probably find it harder than private businesses to demonstrate that each department is autonomous financially and structurally from the parent organization.[81] Finally, managers will err if they do not recognize the "signs" of approaching undue hardship, but they should remember that most reasonable accommodations comprise only about 2 percent of the cost for each employee with HIV/AIDS.[82]

Confidentiality

In both the public and private sectors, HIV/AIDS presents management with two issues concerning the employee rights of privacy and confidentiality. The first issue is narrow in that it deals only with situations involving mandatory HIV antibody blood testing. Here the fundamental question is, who has a right to know the test results? The second, much broader issue deals with employees in the HIV spectrum who seek workplace protections as guaranteed under the Rehab Act and the ADA. The question here is similar to that posed with regard to mandatory testing: who needs to know the HIV status of the employee in order to protect him or her from workplace discrimination? While the first question may be answered by traditional doctrine regarding confidentiality and privacy, the mandate of protection in the Rehab Act and the ADA requires a redefinition of confidentiality and privacy in the age of AIDS.

HIV Test Results

In *Cain v. Hyatt,* the judge observed that "to conclude that persons with AIDS are stigmatized is an understatement; they are widely stereotyped as indelibly miasmic, untouchable, physically and morally polluted."[83]

Given the special stigma attached to HIV/AIDS, the use of mandatory HIV testing as a screening device raises constitutional questions about privacy and confidentiality.[84] Certainly the right to privacy is guaranteed throughout the Bill of Rights.[85] Confidentiality is also guaranteed by the Privacy Act of 1974, which prohibits government from disclosing medical records without the consent of the individual.

The courts have also affirmed the right to confidentiality and privacy. In the *Whalen* and *Thornburgh* cases, the Supreme Court ruled that the collection of a person's health-related information (1) must respect the person's right to confidentiality and (2) must be protected from public disclosure.[86] Given the stigma attached to HIV/AIDS, false or inappropriate reporting can lead to claims of defamation of character. In *Saxton v. Vanzant,* an Ohio court awarded $1.5 million in damages to a worker suspected of having HIV/AIDS when an anonymous note was circulated in the workplace.[87] In the Texas case *Little v. Bryce,* the court sided with the plaintiff in a slander and wrongful discharge case.[88] The employee was falsely accused of having HIV/AIDS. In *Doe v. Borough of Barrington,* a U.S. district court ruled that the city and a police officer were liable to the wife of a person in the HIV spectrum because the police officer disclosed the man's health status to a neighbor.[89] The stigma attached to HIV/AIDS can also lead to claims of psychological stress, as was the case in a 1997 Washington appeals court ruling concerning the state's inability to keep rumors from circulating throughout a community about the HIV status of a prison guard who was bitten by a seropositive inmate.[90] Given the wide range in positive predictive values of HIV antibody test results, as discussed in Appendix B, workplace managers should take seriously the need to maintain the confidentiality of employee health records.

Workplace Protection

When applied to HIV/AIDS situations, the ADA and the Rehab Act have the potential to change the fundamental nature of confidentiality and privacy in the workplace.[91] This capability is one of the many ironies of both federal laws. While each piece of legislation protects the right of confidentiality for disabled employees and job applicants, neither shows how to safeguard it. As noted above, a more traditional view of confidentiality would suggest that a person's HIV status should be communicated only to individuals in the health office of the organization. Also as noted above, the notion of confidentiality traditionally demands that management assume the responsibility for controlling rumors and gossip.

A case-by-case application of either law, however, places management in a quandary with respect to confidentiality, especially when management attempts to provide reasonable accommodations. The effectiveness of accommodation might very well depend on units within the organization. For instance, (1) individuals in human resource management might need to know for purposes of notification and documentation; (2) the legal staff might need to guide management on the application of both laws; (3) the health care office might have to verify HIV infection and develop strategies for responding to case-specific emergencies stemming from both the retrovirus and medication; (4) the insurance staff might be consulted about benefits and to process pharmaceutical claims; (5) the employee assistance program might be called upon to provide counseling and crisis management.

Furthermore, the immediate supervisor will need to be educated about the person's specific disability so that effective and specific reasonable accommodations can be devised. Coworkers may also have to be informed about some functional aspects of the seropositive employee's condition if reasonable accommodation entails rearranging the person's marginal job tasks. Similarly, other supervisors may need to be informed if reasonable accommodations include a job transfer. In addition, a union contract might require union representation in discussions involving job modifications or job transfers.

How many individuals and organization units will need to know something about a person's disability when it comes to providing reasonable accommodations? And to what degree must each person know the many details of the disability? While wrongful disclosure and rumor control will continue to be subjects of litigation, these questions must be answered on a case-by-case basis.[92] As outlined in *Doe v. Septa,* a case involving the right of a self-insured workplace to monitor the use and cost of its health insurance plan, privacy of the employee is not an absolute right; it must always be weighed against the interests of management.[93] In all likelihood, situations involving reasonable accommodation will require greater organizational input and understanding than situations requiring protection from discriminatory acts in the workplace.

One consequence of the Rehab Act and the ADA is thus the need to reinterpret the concepts of privacy and confidentiality. As with issues like reasonable accommodation and undue hardship, this task will certainly entail a case-by-case analysis and will have to be understood and accepted by the individual with HIV/AIDS. Moreover, the search for a new perspective on confidentiality and privacy will have to encompass some of the more traditional components of these concepts, especially in the areas of rumor control. In other words, regardless of how confidentiality looks in a particular situation, coworkers and supervisors will still be prohibited from gossiping about HIV status.

Contact with Others

While employers cannot discriminate against a job applicant or employee in the HIV spectrum, coworkers may express fear and anxiety about working in the same area with that person. An organization may be reminded by unions and non-infected workers alike that the employer is legally liable for the transmission of diseases at the workplace.[94] The National Labor Relations Act, the Labor Management Relations Act (LMRA), and the Occupational Safety and Health Act protect the employee from unsafe and hazardous workplace conditions.[95] Moreover, the courts have long upheld the right of the public to be protected from the spread of diseases.[96]

Fear may lead some employees to consider refusing to work with those in the HIV spectrum.[97] Fear of contact with people who have HIV/AIDS can also affect every aspect of the workplace. Legal scholars, however, agree that "employee refusal must be reasonable and based on a good faith belief of danger to health and safety."[98] In her closing remarks to the jury during an HIV/AIDS-related workplace trial in Cleveland, defense lawyer Denise J. Knecht reminded all that "you are at risk every time you get into your car, every time you walk down the street and every time you go into an operating room. You cannot be risk-free no matter what you do."[99] Furthermore, the LMRA permits the employer to terminate employees who refuse to work if their services are deemed necessary to maintain the organization's operations.[100]

The courts have not ruled recently in favor of workplace arrangements based on the race or gender biases of employees. It is therefore unlikely that either the internal organizational grievance procedures or the American judicial system will permit coworkers to refuse to work in the same environment as individuals in the HIV spectrum.

Because transmission can result only from fluid-to-blood contact, there is no chance of acquiring HIV/AIDS at most public and private workplaces. No one has ever contracted the retrovirus from saliva, nor has anyone ever contracted it from either a pencil wound or a paper cut. In the absence of substantiated evidence about HIV/AIDS-related hazards at the vast majority of workplaces throughout the United States, therefore, employers and coworkers are hard-pressed to find support in the existing legislation and court decisions for refusing to work with individuals in the HIV spectrum. This is also true in "higher-risk" work areas, such as hospital trauma centers and fire departments, because of universal safety precautions mandated by federal and state "occupational safety and health" agencies.

CONCLUSIONS

Job applicants and employees within the HIV spectrum are considered disabled Americans and as such can seek protection under both the Rehab Act and the ADA. This protection is available for both asymptomatic and symptomatic seropositive individuals. The two laws differ in terms of covered entities, affirmative action requirements, enforcement mechanisms, requirements for architectural modifications, and terminology. Job applicants and employees of local government are covered by both pieces of legislation.

Apart from the enumerated differences, the laws are identical. They have the same purpose as well as the same three-pronged definition of disability. Job applicant and employee responsibilities are identical; individuals must empower themselves through notification and documentation requirements to receive both protection and reasonable accommodations. Management's responsibilities are also the same. Managers must understand the essential functions of each job in order to determine whether someone with HIV/AIDS is otherwise qualified for the position. They can employ a variety of screening devices, including HIV antibody blood testing, as long as those devices are narrowly focused, job related, and consistent with business necessity. Managers must also develop reasonable accommodations while understanding where "reasonable" ends and "undue hardship" begins. Confidentiality is certainly protected in the traditional sense when it comes to HIV antibody testing, but the nature of this protection is definitely changing in the search for reasonable accommodations.

Any determination by the employer that an applicant or current employee will not be able to do the job in the future is speculative—even if the person in question has full-blown AIDS. An employer certainly could not refuse to hire an individual on the basis of the applicant's future chances of contracting a form of cancer. The same holds true for people with the retrovirus.

An individual with HIV/AIDS can be terminated from a job only if the person's health places the individual in jeopardy because of the nature of the job or if the person's illnesses jeopardize the health and well-being of others. In most settings, this is not the case. Both the laws and the court decisions typically concur with epidemiological evidence: the overwhelming number of workplaces are deemed "safe" from the threat of contagion.[101] Because there is simply insufficient evidence to suggest that the retrovirus can be transmitted through the course of routine, work-related activities, it is extremely difficult to argue that employees and job applicants in the HIV spectrum pose a hazard to those around them. That coworkers prefer not to want to work with someone who is in the HIV spectrum does not justify either termination of the seropositive individual or refusal to hire in the first place. Such preferences cannot take precedence over the rights of other individuals in the workplace.

The discussion above has several implications. First, most employers in the United States, including local government officials, must be prepared to protect the rights of job applicants and current employees who are in the HIV spectrum. Managers and administrators must guard against discrimination and bias in the workplace, be prepared to provide reasonable accommodations for all seropositive employees, and do so in a variety of ways.

Second, local government managers will be hard-pressed to persuade the courts and others of the need to screen for the retrovirus among job applicants and employees. Regardless of the attitudes and fears of workers, managers, and the community at large, most local government workplaces are simply not at risk, and the essential functions of most jobs do not justify excluding seropositive individuals. Certain positions within the public safety and emergency-response professions may be exceptions to this rule. But even here, local governments that seek to justify screening in these special fields will be better able to withstand judicial scrutiny if they can show that the seropositive individual is unable to perform certain basic job functions or would, in performing them, generate a significant risk of communicating the disease to others.

Third, the courts have been fairly consistent in ruling on behalf of the employee's right to privacy in cases of HIV/AIDS. Local government officials will therefore be expected to uphold the principles of privacy and confidentiality even if members of the community demand that they do otherwise. As far as HIV antibody blood testing is concerned, the citizen's right to know about the workings of government ends where the personnel filing cabinet begins.

Fourth, municipal officials must also begin to redefine the term "confidentiality" so that it better fits the reasonable accommodation requirements of the Rehab Act and the ADA. From the perspective of an effective response to the workplace needs of the individual with HIV/AIDS, knowledge about certain aspects of the infection cannot rest within the walls of the filing cabinet. The fact that each local government may have to assist in developing a constitutionally acceptable new definition of confidentiality may prove the hardest and most challenging workplace task in the age of AIDS.

Fifth, legislation and court decisions also influence the nature of the contact between citizens and public servants in the HIV spectrum that we consider appropriate. Working conditions and workplaces are either safe or unsafe, regardless of the groups involved. Since the courts believe that there is no hazard when noninfected personnel work alongside seropositive employees, it is fair to assume that the same logic and decision rule would be applied to contact with the citizenry. Local government practitioners must therefore be prepared to cope with citizen biases when services are delivered. As with the issue of screening, some public safety and emergency-response workplaces may be targeted as exceptions to the rule. Again, exceptions are most likely to be decided on a case-by-case basis.

Sixth, the law and the courts seem to be encouraging the use of bureaucratic discretion in addressing workplace ramifications of the epidemic. As I have repeatedly noted, much must be determined on a case-by-case basis. Employers have great leeway in making preliminary decisions about the appropriateness of HIV antibody blood testing for all or part of the workforce as well as in establishing voluntary testing programs. Employers have perhaps the greatest discretion in determining what strategies will be used in providing reasonable accommodation. While examples of reasonable accommodation are becoming increasingly abundant, it will remain the responsibility of the administrator to determine initially what is needed and appropriate for both the individual in question and the entire organization.

Finally, the notification and documentation requirements of the Rehab Act and the ADA ironically contribute to the suffering inflicted by the HIV/AIDS epidemic. While self-disclosure is the price of protection, the social stigma attached to the retrovirus makes it extremely difficult for many individuals to stand up and empower themselves. The situation is exacerbated by the absence of readily apparent and uniquely shared characteristics that could help HIV-challenged individuals to identify each other and to derive strength, courage, and support from knowing that they are not alone. This constitutes a situation that might be called the Rosa Parks dilemma. On the one hand, the seropositive individual must assert her rights just as Rosa Parks so bravely did on the bus in Montgomery, Alabama. Yet unlike Rosa Parks, the seropositive individual must do so in a relative vacuum, not knowing who else she can count on as a result of sharing membership in this particular protected group. Hence, self-disclosure remains a tough decision: whether to be a Rosa Parks in the workplace or simply remain silent and fundamentally unprotected. For both the job applicant and the employee with HIV/AIDS, therefore, empowerment creates a special climate of risk as well as the only hope of security.

4

Attitudes toward HIV/AIDS in the Workplace

As we have seen, management must support each job applicant and employee with HIV/AIDS while simultaneously protecting the organization from undue hardship. The present chapter analyzes the attitudes of local government chief administrative officers (CAOs)—city managers and mayors—toward this challenge and others surrounding HIV/AIDS and the workplace. In doing so, it reexamines from the CAO's vantage point the concerns introduced in Chapter 2. Do officials think that local government is sufficiently prepared to deal with the workplace ramifications of HIV/AIDS? What do city managers and mayors believe about direct, work-related contact between seropositive employees and citizens? What are CAOs' opinions about HIV antibody blood testing of the workforce? What are their views on the issue of confidentiality? How do municipal CAOs view the issues of reasonable accommodation and undue hardship? Have the attitudes of city managers and mayors changed between the late 1980s and the mid-1990s?

ATTITUDES AND POLICY IMPLEMENTATION

Attitudes help determine how and when a public problem will be solved. One needs only to remember any of a multitude of events in recent history to appreciate the impact that public opinion can have on policy outcomes. Public opinion in the early 1940s affirmed the government's decision to intern many Japanese-Americans—and ironically, public opinion of the 1990s spurred the federal government's decision to apologize and compensate the internees for violating their constitutional rights. Changing views of the citizenry also influenced public policies about the civil rights of people of color and women during the 1960s and 1970s. A growing public awareness of, and sense of urgency about, the HIV/AIDS epidemic is also changing public policies. In the 1990s, changes in attitudes led to citizen-appointed boards being created to advise policymakers about the many ramifications of the retrovirus and the needs of its victims.

Attitudes of key administrators typically play an informal yet significant role in the design and implementation of programs mandated to address specific problems.[1] While this statement is true at all levels of government, the attitudes of municipal practitioners are particularly important in a federal system that lacks strong and constant monitoring mechanisms at the national and state levels. The ability of the judicial and regulatory systems to oversee local government practices is also limited. While specific cases may be referred for independent administrative review and adjustment of practices, officials are not present to monitor the consequences of every personnel decision that takes place daily in every workplace throughout the nation. For the most part, therefore, no external agency can continually enforce compliance with every federal and state law.[2] Until a specific complaint is filed, the environment is presumed consistent with both the letter and the spirit of the law.

The attitudes of city managers and mayors are more critical in implementing controversial and perhaps locally unpopular laws.[3] Supervisors and employees have a choice to make. On the one hand, the political costs of compliance may sometimes seem to outweigh the legal and ethical benefits of compliance. Some local government practitioners may therefore decide not to implement unpopular policies—they may refuse outright or simply fail to do so. At the other extreme, employees' and supervisors' positive attitudes on a controversial issue may make the adoption of distasteful regulations and practices seem more palatable.

The attitudes of CAOs particularly influence the workplace ramifications of HIV/AIDS. While the Rehab Act and the ADA are designed to protect disabled individuals from workplace discrimination, the nature of the HIV/AIDS epidemic complicates the task. As with other controversial issues, CAOs may be soured by the politics of the retrovirus. Given the prejudice that can accompany HIV/AIDS, city managers and mayors may perceive a risk to their careers if they assist members of the protected group in the face of opposition from key sources of political support within the workplace hierarchy and throughout the community.

On the other hand, CAOs whose opinions are free from politics and bigotry can positively influence city hall's response with respect to two interconnected tasks: meeting the job-related needs of members of the disabled group and building a workplace environment that encourages and supports the self-disclosure required by both acts.

Each city manager or mayor can choose to avoid the law, simply implement the letter of the law, or take additional positive steps in assisting job applicants and employees in the HIV spectrum. CAOs can also choose whether or not to express their views on this subject within staff meetings, through memoranda to the workforce, and in informal and formal forums throughout the community. Their views will affect their decision.

For all of these reasons, practitioners' attitudes about HIV/AIDS are crucial in setting both tone and practice within the workplace. As Frank J. Thompson once observed, "Those who recruit, fire, allocate positions, and so on may be bureaucrats but they are not simple cogs in the machine. Often they have significant leeway to choose among various courses of action."[4] This statement is particularly true with HIV/AIDS. How the city manager or mayor feels about the epidemic might well supply the initial answer to such questions as how "reasonable" is reasonable accommodation or how "nondiscriminatory" is nondiscrimination. City leaders clearly have the power to construct either a responsive and caring environment or one colored by misunderstandings, bigotry, and hostility.

PRACTITIONERS' ATTITUDES

I analyzed the opinions of local government practitioners using a four-page questionnaire, included in Appendix A, that consists of seventy-eight items assessing workplace attitudes, organization practices and policies, and background information about the respondent CAO. It is similar to the survey instrument used six years earlier in the first edition of this book, but it includes additional items pertinent to the issues of reasonable accommodation and undue hardship. As with the original survey instrument, I minimized response bias by randomizing the order of items within category (attitude and practice) and by stating approximately half of the items in the negative.[5] As with the original questionnaire, the validity of this survey instrument was strengthened by modifications made after a pretest had been sent to a variety of practitioners, HIV/AIDS experts, and academicians.

A systematic random sample of 971 communities, each with a population of 2,000 or more, was drawn from a list provided by the International City and County Management Association.[6] Identification numbers were used to track returns. Up to four first-class mailings went to the CAO of each community during the winter months of 1993–1994. Questionnaires were mailed at four- to six-week intervals (but not during weeks with holidays). Each envelope included a cover letter, the author's business card, a copy of the questionnaire, and a prepaid business reply envelope.[7]

A total of 520 CAOs, 54 percent of the sample, responded to the survey: 51 percent were mayors, and 49 percent were city managers.[8] The average respondent was a European-American male of middle age who was well educated.[9] The overwhelming majority of CAOs hold moderate to conservative political views; only a few claimed to be either very liberal or very conservative.[10] The CAOs represent communities from all states, with an average population of 107,000.[11] Most CAOs consider their communities to be in either rural or suburban settings.[12] These factors attest to the representativeness of the sample and to its comparability to the responses from the original survey.

Understanding the ADA and HIV/AIDS

The responses of municipal government CAOs yield insight into their general views and level of understanding about the ADA and HIV/AIDS. As table 7 shows, the findings are somewhat mixed. While the majority of CAOs believe that they are knowledgeable about the ADA (item 1), nearly 20 percent remain uncertain. Although over half of the respondents say that they are sufficiently knowledgeable about how to handle HIV/AIDS-related situations, nearly 30 percent are not sure (item 2). The majority of CAOs, however, believe that current procedures are in-

Table 7. Understanding the ADA and HIV/AIDS: Questionnaire Response
(percent)

Questionnaire Item	Strongly Disagree	Disagree	Neutral/ Undecided	Agree	Strongly Agree
Item 1					
I am sufficiently knowledgeable about the ADA to handle disability-related situations in the workplace. (n = 516)	3.3	11.7	18.1	49.5	17.5
Item 2					
I am sufficiently knowledgeable about HIV/ AIDS to handle HIV/ AIDS-related situations in the workplace. (n = 518)	2.3	18.0	28.8	42.5	8.5
Item 3					
City policies are adequate for handling HIV/AIDS-related situations at work. (n = 514)	12.5	45.5	23.0	16.5	2.5
Item 4					
In my city government, there is need to develop specific plans and procedures for dealing with HIV/AIDS in the workplace. (n = 514)	1.6	14.6	24.3	48.2	11.3

sufficient to handle HIV/AIDS-related situations in the workplace (item 3), and
they see a need to develop better policies and plans (item 4). Approximately one-
quarter of the CAOs are uncertain about the adequacy of current procedures (item
3) and the need for specific HIV/AIDS plans for the workplace (item 4).

The findings in table 8 tap the CAOs' application of knowledge about HIV/
AIDS to workplace situations and, in doing so, provide insight into the workplace
environment. The results indicate that, even in the 1990s, fairly well-educated people
may lack understanding about the epidemiology of HIV/AIDS. While over 85 percent of the CAOs know that HIV/AIDS is not transmitted casually (item 1), just

Table 8. Understanding the Epidemiology of HIV/AIDS: Questionnaire
Response (percent)

Questionnaire Item	Strongly Disagree	Disagree	Neutral/ Undecided	Agree	Strongly Agree
Item 1					
You cannot catch HIV/AIDS from casual contact with people who have HIV/AIDS. (n = 515)	0.6	1.6	11.3	58.1	28.5
Item 2					
It's OK for employees with HIV/AIDS to have direct contact with citizens. (n = 517)	3.9	10.8	29.8	42.7	12.8
Item 3					
It's OK for employees with HIV/AIDS to have direct contact with children. (n = 515)	4.4	17.7	30.5	39.8	7.6

over half believe that it is "OK" for city employees with HIV/AIDS to have direct contact with citizens (item 2). The number of city managers and mayors who are either uncertain about, or disagree with, direct contact between HIV/AIDS employees and the public increases when such contact involves the children of the community (item 3).

CAO wariness about contact between HIV/AIDS-challenged employees and people in the community may also stem from political factors rather than simply from lack of epidemiological understanding. The findings reported in table 9 perhaps reflect these political considerations. Given the stigma often attached to HIV/AIDS, it is not surprising that most city managers and mayors believe that voters would likely oppose the hiring of individuals in the HIV spectrum (item 1). This concern is felt although fewer than 10 percent report that similar fears have been expressed by members of city council (item 2).

Applying the ADA in the Workplace

Table 10 examines CAO attitudes toward the rights of employees with HIV/AIDS. Here the items are separated into two categories: supportive and nonsupportive views. Again, the findings are somewhat mixed.

Table 9. Perceptions About Citizens' Attitudes and City Council
Concerns: Questionnaire Response (percent)

Questionnaire Item	Strongly Disagree	Disagree	Neutral/ Undecided	Agree	Strongly Agree
Item 1					
Most citizens in my community would oppose the hiring of people with HIV/AIDS to the city's workforce. (n = 517)	1.7	8.7	28.0	45.3	16.2
Item 2					
City council has expressed concern about the possibility of having people with HIV/AIDS employed on the city's workforce.[a] (n = 503)	—	93.2	—	6.8	—

[a] For item 2, "disagree" was no and "agree" was yes.

The vast majority of CAOs believe that employees with HIV/AIDS should be treated like other city workers (item 1) and that seropositive employees have a right to continue to work as long as health conditions allow (item 2). Only about half of the city managers and mayors believe that it is okay to hire people with HIV/AIDS (item 3), however, and less than a majority agree that these employees should be protected by the ADA (item 4).[13]

Most city managers and mayors believe it wrong to discriminate against employees with HIV/AIDS (item 5). But the number of CAOs who are undecided rises dramatically when they are asked to consider important workplace issues, such as the segregation of seropositive employees from the rest of the workforce (18.4 percent, item 6) and the termination of employees with "full-blown" AIDS regardless of ability to perform essential job functions (21.8 percent, item 7). The fact that approximately 85 percent of city managers and mayors believe that employees with HIV/AIDS should not be discharged from the workforce still leaves a substantial proportion (about 15 percent) of municipalities with CAOs who are either uncertain or in disagreement with such employment practices (item 8).

Table 11 shows three questionnaire items that are designed to measure the level of knowledge about federal guidelines on reasonable accommodation as applied to situations involving HIV/AIDS. Each item represents a different scenario. The first item might involve a person with an AIDS-related opportunistic disease or cancer

Table 10. Attitudes About People with HIV/AIDS in the Workplace: Questionnaire Response of Chief Administrative Officers (percent)

Questionnaire Item	Strongly Disagree	Disagree	Neutral/ Undecided	Agree	Strongly Agree
Supportive Attitudes					
Item 1					
As long as city employees with HIV/AIDS are able to perform the essential functions or tasks of a job, they should be treated the same as other city employees. (n = 518)	1.7	4.8	9.7	56.0	27.8
Item 2					
A city employee with HIV/AIDS has a right to continue to work as long as his/her health condition allows. (n = 516)	0.4	4.1	8.9	64.7	21.9
Item 3					
It is OK to hire people with HIV/AIDS. (n = 519)	6.6	13.9	23.7	37.8	18.1
Item 4					
People with HIV/AIDS should be protected by the ADA. (n = 514)	6.4	19.6	27.8	30.9	15.2
Nonsupportive Attitudes					
Item 5					
It should be OK to discriminate against city employees who have HIV/AIDS. (n = 515)	36.3	50.9	8.5	3.7	0.6
Item 6					
City employees with HIV/AIDS should be separated from other employees. (n = 516)	10.9	61.2	18.4	6.6	2.9

Table 10. continued

Questionnaire Item	Strongly Disagree	Disagree	Neutral/ Undecided	Agree	Strongly Agree
Item 7					
Employees with full-blown AIDS should be terminated from the workplace, regardless of their ability to do their job. (n = 519)	23.9	44.3	21.8	7.3	2.7
Item 8					
City employees with HIV/AIDS should be discharged from the city workforce. (n = 516)	29.1	55.4	10.5	4.1	1.0

who requires reasonable accommodations so that the job's essential functions can be performed. The second item might involve a person who is seropositive but remains asymptomatic. The third item might involve a person with a record of having an AIDS-related opportunistic disease or cancer, but the condition is temporarily in remission. As noted in Chapter 3, both the Rehab Act and the ADA protect people who find themselves in any of these three situations and require work organizations to provide reasonable accommodations.

The opinions of the nation's city managers and mayors, reported in table 11, further underscore an absence of understanding about the application of the Rehab Act and the ADA to workplace situations involving people with HIV/AIDS. Nearly two-thirds of the CAOs are either uncertain about, or disagree with, the prospects of providing reasonable accommodations to people with HIV/AIDS (item 1). More than three out of every four respondents do not agree with the prospect of providing reasonable accommodations to people with HIV/AIDS when no physical symptoms are present (item 2) or when such symptoms are in remission (item 3).

Table 12 reports the attitudes of city managers and mayors toward the issue of undue hardship. More than two-thirds of the CAOs are apprehensive about the cost of reasonable accommodations for employees with HIV/AIDS (item 1). This concern may have to do more with budgets than with anything else, since over 70 percent of the CAOs are also worried about the cost of providing reasonable accommodations for any disabled employee, regardless of the type or nature of disability (item 2).

Table 11. Attitudes Toward Reasonable Accommodations for Employees with HIV/AIDS: Questionnaire Response of Chief Administrative Officers (percent)

Questionnaire Item	Strongly Disagree	Disagree	Neutral/ Undecided	Agree	Strongly Agree
Item 1 City employees with HIV/AIDS should be given special assistance or accommodation so that they can perform their job's essential functions or basic tasks. (n = 517)	4.8	32.7	27.9	30.0	4.6
Item 2 City employees who have HIV/AIDS, but have no physical symptoms or conditions, should be given special assistance or accommodation in the workplace. (n = 517)	12.0	45.6	19.1	19.5	3.7
Item 3 City employees with HIV/AIDS should receive special assistance or accommodation at the workplace when illnesses are in remission. (n = 514)	3.7	49.2	27.8	16.5	2.7

Testing and Confidentiality

Table 13 reports the views of city managers and mayors on the subject of HIV antibody testing of the workforce. With the exception of testing suspected homosexuals (item 1), which less than 10 percent support, local government practitioners seem evenly divided on this issue. Approximately 50 percent of the respondents oppose mandatory testing of the workforce (item 2) and oppose mandatory blood testing for new employees (item 3). Similarly, almost 50 percent of the CAOs oppose mandatory HIV antibody blood testing for persons who have direct contact with

Table 12. Attitudes About Undue Hardship: Questionnaire Response of Chief
Administrative Officers (percent)

Questionnaire Item	Strongly Disagree	Disagree	Neutral/ Undecided	Agree	Strongly Agree
Item 1					
In most cases, it will be too expensive to provide special workplace assistance or accommodation to city employees who have HIV/AIDS. (n = 515)	3.7	30.1	38.1	24.1	4.1
Item 2					
Providing special assistance or accommodation to disabled workers will lead to the city having to cut budgets in other areas. (n = 516)	4.7	22.5	27.7	37.6	7.6

the public. The "neutral/undecided" category in items 2–4, however, comprises approximately 25 percent of all responses on the issue of screening.

Table 14 reports the views of practitioners about confidentiality in the workplace. City managers and mayors tend to respect the right of confidentiality of the worker, especially in the area of health and medical records. While two-thirds of the CAOs believe that the laws should allow the city to collect information about employees' health status (item 1), more than 80 percent believe that blood test results ought to remain confidential (item 2) and more than 70 percent believe that the employee's health condition is personal and confidential (item 3). Nearly 95 percent of the practitioners agree that it is the city's responsibility to protect medical information collected about workers (item 4).

As reported in table 14, most practitioners also believe that the employee's right of confidentiality outweighs the right of the citizen to know about the presence of the retrovirus in the workplace. Approximately 63 percent of the respondents think that citizens do not have the right to know the identity of municipal workers who are in the HIV spectrum (item 5). More than two-thirds of the CAOs also believe that citizens do not have the right to know the number of employees with the retrovirus (item 6), and over 55 percent say that citizens do not have the right to know which departments have employees with HIV/AIDS (item 7).

Table 13. Views on HIV/AIDS Testing: Questionnaire Response of Local Government Officials (percent)

Questionnaire Item	Strongly Disagree	Disagree	Neutral/ Undecided	Agree	Strongly Agree
Item 1					
Mandatory blood testing for suspected homosexuals (n = 518)	36.2	45.7	9.8	5.4	2.9
Item 2					
Mandatory blood testing for all employees (n = 516)	10.1	40.3	23.1	20.3	6.2
Item 3					
Mandatory blood testing for new employees (n = 518)	13.9	37.5	25.5	17.2	6.0
Item 4					
Mandatory blood testing for workers with direct contact with the public (n = 516)	10.3	38.8	27.9	18.6	4.5

CHANGES IN ATTITUDE

It has been six years since CAOs responded to the survey reported in the first edition of this book. In terms of the socialization process, six years typically do not constitute a length of time during which adults' fundamental attitudes and behavior would likely change and particularly not in professions like local government management, where incumbents risk losing their jobs if they promote rapid change. Most city managers and mayors choose not to be ahead of the curve in their own communities, especially when it comes to policies with controversial social and political consequences.

Still, six years is a long time in terms of increases in the HIV/AIDS knowledge base and public awareness. HIV/AIDS education in the 1990s is more sophisticated than it was in the 1980s, and the results are more widespread in society. As noted in Chapter 1, stereotypes have changed as famous people have publicly announced their HIV status and as the number of people with HIV/AIDS in every community has increased. Most people now know someone who is in the HIV spectrum, whether or not they know about his or her HIV status. The passage of the ADA has also made people more aware of the rights of persons with HIV/AIDS.

Table 14. Views about Confidentiality of HIV/AIDS in the Workplace:
Questionnaire Response of Chief Administrative Officers (percent)

Questionnaire Item	Strongly Disagree	Disagree	Neutral/ Undecided	Agree	Strongly Agree
Item 1					
Laws should allow the city to collect information regarding a city employee's health condition. (n = 515)	3.3	11.7	18.1	49.5	17.5
Item 2					
City workers have the right to keep AIDS blood tests confidential. (n = 519)	0.8	5.6	12.5	46.2	34.9
Item 3					
Worker's health condition is personal and confidential. (n = 519)	4.2	13.9	10.2	39.5	32.2
Item 4					
The city must protect medical information collected about workers. (n = 519)	0.4	1.2	3.7	47.8	47.0
Item 5					
Citizens have the right to know the identity of HIV/AIDS workers. (n =517)	22.6	40.8	20.9	12.8	2.9
Item 6					
Citizens have the right to know the number of HIV/AIDS city employees. (n = 516)	20.2	47.5	19.4	11.2	1.7
Item 7					
Citizens have the right to know which departments have HIV/AIDS workers. (n = 519)	16.4	39.9	21.8	15.4	6.6

Have the attitudes of city managers and mayors changed over the past six years? Table 15 sheds some light on this question. More CAOs say that they are knowledgeable about HIV/AIDS, but there is also a slight increase in the number who remain uncertain about the subject (item 1). There is a substantial increase in understanding that citizens cannot contract HIV/AIDS from normal interactions with infected employees, although the numbers of CAOs who are still uncertain on this issue also remains high (item 2). The findings reported in item 3 suggest that there is little change in opinion about the level of local government preparedness in dealing with the workplace ramifications of HIV/AIDS. Perhaps partly because of increased awareness of the retrovirus, however, there appears to be a growing recognition of the need for the adoption of HIV/AIDS plans for the workplace (item 4).

Have the views of city managers and mayors changed about mandatory testing and confidentiality? To some extent, item 5 and item 6 suggest that they have. Substantially fewer CAOs support mandatory HIV testing for employees with direct contact with the citizenry, although there is a slight increase in the number who are uncertain. There also continues to be substantial opposition to letting citizens know which employees have HIV/AIDS, although about one in five of the CAOs remain undecided on this issue, too.

What about CAO attitudes toward the workplace rights of people with HIV/AIDS? Item 7 and item 8 suggest that opinions remain mixed. Overwhelming support on the "right to work" issue remains in the 1990s and in fact continues to grow. Support for the right of employees with HIV/AIDS to have access to reasonable accommodations has grown somewhat since the late 1980s but still remains significantly low, given the law of the land. In fact, almost the same number of mayors and city managers were uncertain in both surveys on the critical issue of reasonable accommodation.

CONCLUSIONS

Do the attitudes and opinions of local government CAOs reflect a belief that they are prepared to deal with the workplace ramifications of HIV/AIDS? The answer seems to be no. Overall, there appears to be general understanding of the ADA but insufficient understanding of its application to workplace situations involving HIV/AIDS. CAOs express mixed and uncertain views about the acceptability of seropositive individuals in the workplace.

Are city managers and mayors comfortable with the prospect that employees with HIV/AIDS will have contact with citizens, including children? Many practitioners express concern about such interaction, and they are concerned about the public reaction to having people with HIV/AIDS employed by city government. In the minds of some CAOs, solutions to real and potential workplace situations pertaining to HIV/AIDS may lie in the shadow of anticipated community response as well as in the light of epidemiology and law.

Table 15. Comparison of CAO Attitudes, 1989 and 1994 (percent)

	1989		1994	
Questionnaire Item	Agree/ Supportive[a]	Neutral/ Undecided	Agree/ Supportive[b]	Neutral/ Undecided
Item 1 Have sufficient knowl- edge about HIV/AIDS	36.8	24.1	51.0	28.8
Item 2 It's OK for HIV/AIDS workers to have direct con- tact with children	34.8	29.7	47.4	30.5
Item 3 City's policies are ade- quate to handle HIV/ AIDS	20.1	21.4	19.0	23.0
Item 4 Need for specific HIV/AIDS plan	52.2	24.3	59.5	24.3
Item 5 Mandatory testing for em- ployees with contact with citizens	33.2	24.6	23.1	27.9
Item 6 Citizens have a right to know the identity of worker with HIV/AIDS	17.9	17.3	15.7	20.9
Item 7 Workers with HIV/ AIDS have a right to work as long as their health con- ditions allow	71.9	16.6	86.6	8.9
Item 8 Reasonable accommoda- tions for employees with HIV/AIDS	24.1	24.3	34.6	27.9

[a] For purposes of this table, the Likert scale has been collapsed: agree/supportive = 5 + 6 + 7.

[b] For purposes of this table, the Likert scale has been collapsed: agree/supportive = 4 + 5.

CAOs are unsure as to whether mandatory policies on HIV antibody blood testing should be implemented. While most disagree with mandatory testing, this issue seems to generate the most dissent and uncertainty among city managers and mayors. Most agree, however, that test results and other medical evidence should remain confidential. City managers and mayors believe that the worker's right of confidentiality exceeds the citizen's right to know about the existence of the retrovirus in the workplace. Should employees with HIV/AIDS have access to reasonable accommodations at the workplace? Here the answer is mixed at best.

A comparison of responses to the two surveys suggests that wider understanding and support exists for employees with HIV/AIDS in the mid-1990s, but the level of support remains marginal. Three patterns continue to hold: (1) practitioners support general issues concerning HIV/AIDS and the rights of seropositive workers; (2) support declines when the topic turns to specific issues, such as reasonable accommodation, citizen contact, and HIV screening; and (3) there is substantial uncertainty on all issues pertaining to the workplace in the age of AIDS.

In short, at the time when they need it most, individuals within the HIV spectrum cannot count on practitioners to create a supportive environment or even to comply with federal legislation. Therefore, in addition to fighting the retrovirus inside their bodies, PLWAs may have to fight fear and ignorance about HIV/AIDS inside the workplace. Seropositive workers who face either hostility or indifference should recognize the need to choose between hiding their health conditions as long as possible and accepting the primary responsibility for securing workplace assistance and guarantees against discriminatory practices. The fact that each employee with HIV/AIDS may believe that he or she is the only one in the workforce who is seropositive—central to the Rosa Parks dilemma—may make the choice of empowerment through self-disclosure harder. Each person's ability to confront a nonsupportive workplace environment will also depend upon the progress of the retrovirus. Many workers with HIV/AIDS may prefer to forgo the battle.

The findings paint a rather bleak picture of preparedness in the municipal government workplace. Still, while city managers and mayors may not understand how to apply federal legislation to situations involving people with HIV/AIDS, survey findings do not portray them as suffering from "AIDS-phobia." It is clear, however, that many find themselves in a genuine quandary. They want to do what is right for all concerned parties: employees in the HIV spectrum, other employees, the municipality, the citizenry, and their own careers. But what are the right steps to take? That HIV/AIDS continues to spread, and is still not seen as affecting all segments of the community, makes it even harder than usual to determine what is right.

5

Workplace Policies and Procedures

LOCAL GOVERNMENT PREPAREDNESS, as we have seen, is the extent to which policies and procedures have been developed to manage HIV/AIDS in the workplace. This chapter considers preparedness and explores the impact of various forces in effecting the adoption of HIV/AIDS programs and procedures. The findings here are based on the survey instrument and methodology that were described in the preface and in Chapter 4.

CONCEPTUAL FRAMEWORK

The issue to be explained, or the dependent variable, is local government preparedness. In the context of the emergency management perspective introduced in Chapter 2, "preparedness" can be defined as the extent to which municipalities are ready to respond. In managing various types of public emergencies, practitioners rely on four basic steps or processes:

Step 1: Mitigation
Deciding what to do when a crisis or emergency has been identified.

Step 2: Preparedness
Developing a response plan and training first responders to deal effectively with the situation.

Step 3: Response
Implementing the emergency plan. Providing assistance to those affected by the crisis.

Step 4: Recovery
Providing support to facilitate the resumption of normal activities.[1]

In this study, "local government preparedness" encompasses all activities through step 2 in the emergency management process. Regardless of the current health status of the workforce, local government is considered prepared to handle the workplace ramifications of HIV/AIDS if it has determined what needs to be done in the event that personnel contract the retrovirus and if it has actually developed and implemented a strategy or response plan for dealing with that situation.

What forces affect levels of preparedness among municipalities in coping with HIV/AIDS in the work force? Three sets of factors, or independent variables, can play substantial roles in determining the nature and extent of organizational responsiveness: (1) personal characteristics of CAOs, (2) the organization's environment, and (3) the organizational experience.[2]

The effect of the first independent variable, personal characteristics of decision makers, has been examined in a wide variety of studies. We sometimes forget that organizations consist of people and that people determine the organizational culture. While workplace cultures are in large part historically based and predetermined, it remains true that "leaders influence the development and expression of culture in their organizations."[3] Leaders can help sustain or modify existing cultures, and they can use their positions to transform the workplace environment into something completely different. Within the work setting, therefore, CAOs have the power to initiate changes that can lead to differences in organizational attitude and behavior.

The role played by individuals in shaping organizational responses is also noted throughout the policy implementation literature.[4] Within the framework of American federalism, the best-laid plans of Washington can be either accomplished or thwarted by actions and nonactions—formal and informal behavior—of people in Boston or Bakersfield, especially in the case of antidiscrimination policies, such as those involving school desegregation or the integration of a protected group into the workforce.[5] Previous research dealing with affirmative action policies suggests that factors such as issue-specific attitudes and general political values that are congruent with the law and a clear understanding of the policy to be implemented can contribute to effective policy implementation.[6] Moreover, key administrators who are older and better educated tend to be more successful at implementing affirmative action policies.[7] The personal backgrounds of city managers and mayors, therefore, should affect their level of preparedness to deal with the workplace ramifications of HIV/AIDS.

The second factor or independent variable is the organization's environment, including background demographics, local politics, and the form or structure of government. It is important to look at the demographics, or unique community characteristics, because these may prove to be influential in shaping the nature of responses.

Previous studies show that, while differences tend to be a matter of degree and not necessarily direction, urban/rural distinctions may influence city hall.[8] The complexities of the urban environment, some argue, make the tasks of local government truly unique.[9] In contrast to their rural counterparts, municipal government personnel in urban areas tend to have greater expertise and are able to assert greater specialization in dealing with a wider variety of problems.[10] Urban governments also tend to make greater use of sophisticated management tools to increase their responsive capacity.[11] Rural local governments, on the other hand, tend to have fewer resources and less flexibility in responding to the needs of their citizenry.[12] Unlike their urban counterparts, local government professionals in rural settings tend to have fewer opportunities to pool resources.

Research also shows that the size of the community, as well as urban-rural environmental distinctions, can influence local government decision-making processes and outcomes.[13] Issues of great concern seem to be articulated more thoroughly and readily, and remedies sought more promptly, in cities that have a critical mass of both people and experiences.[14] Given that the HIV/AIDS epidemic is currently most pronounced in larger cities, the need for preparedness is greater in these areas than in smaller cities and towns. It is certainly a topic of greater visibility in larger cities than elsewhere. The size and setting of the community, or the nature of the community, may prove significant in determining the level and quality of organizational responsiveness.[15]

It is also important to examine the political dimension, which helps shape actions and nonactions taken by organizations within the task environment.[16] Nicholas Henry reminds us that this is particularly true in the case of public organizations, where the environment tends to be more "complex, aggressive and intrusive" than in the private sector.[17] The external dimension may prove to be even more important for organizations trying to deal with HIV/AIDS, given the political and inaccurate nature of HIV/AIDS information that is often found throughout the task environment.[18] What a local government does in its workplace, especially in situations involving HIV/AIDS, may well be shaped by the prevailing views and political forces within the community.

One final aspect of the second independent variable, the organization's environment, deals with the structure of government within which the organization operates. Here we focus on municipal organizations using either the council-manager or mayor-council forms of government. In comparison to mayors, the literature suggests that city managers tend to be more businesslike, placing greater emphasis on having efficiently run organizations and showing more interest in searching for innovative solutions to organizational problems.[19] While city managers seem to be more concerned with the internal operations of city hall, mayors tend to place greater weight on responding to the external political environment.[20] That is, mayors seem to demonstrate greater concern about community-based forces and the reaction of these forces to the delivery of services than do their counterparts in council-manager governments.

Previous research suggests that structure may help shape the actions of local government but leaves the direction of impact open for further examination. For instance, city managers may demonstrate greater preparedness to deal with HIV/AIDS-related workplace conditions because such conditions threaten the efficiency of the organization. Mayors, on the other hand, may be better prepared to manage HIV/AIDS-related situations when the ramifications become a concern either to key groups in the community or to the voter at large.

The third independent variable focuses on the organizational experience in dealing with HIV/AIDS. Herbert A. Simon reminds us that an organization's memory of past experiences can influence its approach to solving a problem in the future.[21] Empirical studies tend to verify Simon's observation. Whether in the service delivery area or in its internal workings, how an organization responds to a situation is more often than not a function of previous experience in the matter.[22] In the case of technological or natural disasters, local governments experienced in dealing with similar crises will tend to be better prepared, to be more responsive, and to use fewer resources than those with no experience.[23] Dealing with the many facets of HIV/AIDS can produce great frustration and anxiety in many organizations, but such experience can also present vast opportunities.[24] Organizations may become more responsive as they begin to acquire additional firsthand experience in managing HIV/AIDS-related situations in the workplace. Such experience may help reshape the organization's practices toward employees and job applicants in the HIV spectrum.

The conceptual framework is illustrated schematically in figure 1, which shows three factors contributing to municipal preparedness: (1) personal characteristics of CAOs, including attitudes, knowledge base, and background attributes; (2) the environment of municipal government, including community characteristics, local politics, and the structure or form of government; and (3) the organization's experience with dealing with HIV/AIDS-related situations in the workplace.

OPERATIONALIZATION

Dependent and independent variables were operationalized by items incorporated in the questionnaire (see Appendix A). The dependent variable local government preparedness was measured in four ways. First, each respondent was asked if his or her municipality had adopted a set of formal procedures for dealing with HIV/AIDS-related situations. This indicator of the dependent variable will be called "HIV/AIDS Plan."

Second, because local government practitioners may address workplace consequences of the retrovirus without actually having developed a comprehensive HIV/AIDS plan, they were also asked whether disparate procedures and policies are in place to assist workers in the HIV spectrum. This indicator, "HIV/AIDS Workplace Assistance," was composed of the following questionnaire items:

- Provides disability retirement
- Provides for voluntary HIV antibody blood testing
- Provides a specialist to handle all issues pertaining to the ADA
- Ensures the investigation of complaints about HIV/AIDS-related discrimination

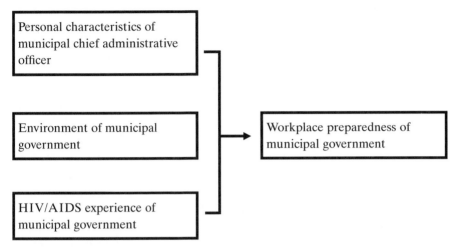

Figure 1. Conceptual Framework for Empirical Analysis of Workplace Preparedness

- Provides HIV/AIDS employees with benefit consultation to assist in the management of health, leave, and other benefits
- Refers employees concerned about having caught HIV/AIDS to agencies that offer supportive services
- Provides information about HIV/AIDS to employees
- Provides information to employees about the ADA
- Provides HIV/AIDS education to employees
- Provides training for supervisors on how to deal with employees with HIV/AIDS[25]

The other two indicators of the dependent variable tapped municipal government's preparedness to provide "reasonable accommodations for employees with HIV/AIDS" and "reasonable accommodations for job applicants with HIV/AIDS." Questionnaire items for both dependent variables were the following:

- Makes workplace accommodations similar to those made for people with other disabilities
- Modifies work schedules to meet the workplace needs of persons with HIV/AIDS
- Restructures jobs to meet the workplace needs of persons with HIV/AIDS
- Acquires or modifies equipment to meet the workplace needs of persons with HIV/AIDS
- Provides qualified readers or interpreters to meet the workplace needs of persons with HIV/AIDS
- Modifies tests to meet the workplace needs of persons with HIV/AIDS

- Modifies training materials to meet the workplace needs of persons with HIV/AIDS
- Transfers them to other work areas if persons with HIV/AIDS request such transfers
- Pays for all necessary workplace assistance or accommodations[26]

Survey items were also used to measure indicators of the three independent variables: CAO personal characteristics, the organization's environment, and the workplace experience with HIV/AIDS.[27] The CAO personal characteristics of "supportive workplace attitudes" and "nonsupportive workplace attitudes," checked for multicollinearity, were measured by creating two independent scales from two groups of survey items.[28]

Supportive Attitudes

Item 1: As long as city employees with HIV/AIDS are able to perform the essential functions or tasks of a job, they should be treated the same as other city employees.

Item 2: A city employee with HIV/AIDS has a right to continue to work as long as his/her health condition allows.

Item 3: It is OK to hire people with HIV/AIDS.

Item 4: People with HIV/AIDS should be protected by the ADA.

Nonsupportive Attitudes

Item 5: It should be OK to discriminate against city employees who have HIV/AIDS.

Item 6: City employees with HIV/AIDS should be separated from other employees.

Item 7: Employees with full-blown AIDS should be terminated from the workplace, regardless of their ability to do their job.

Item 8: City employees with HIV/AIDS should be discharged from the city workforce.

The indicator, "attitudes toward reasonable accommodation," was also measured by forming a scale out of survey items.

Item 1: City employees with HIV/AIDS should be given special assistance or accommodation so that they can perform their job's essential functions or basic tasks.

Item 2: City employees who have HIV/AIDS, but have no physical symptoms or conditions, should be given special assistance or accommodation in the workplace.

Item 3: City employees with HIV/AIDS should receive special assistance or accommodation at the workplace when illnesses are in remission.

Table 16. Internal Consistency of Dependent Variable Scales and Independent
Variable Scales

Variable	Cronbach's Alpha
Workplace assistance activities	0.76
Reasonable accommodation for employees with HIV/AIDS	0.89
Reasonable accommodation for job applicants with HIV/AIDS	0.90
Supportive workplace attitudes[a]	0.63
Nonsupportive workplace attitudes[a]	0.60
Attitudes toward reasonable accommodation[a]	0.67

[a] While these scores are somewhat lower than the scores for the dependent variable scales, they are still in the range of acceptability. For examples of Cronbach's alpha of similar magnitude, see Dennis Daly, "Merit Pay Enters with a Whimper: The Initial Federal Civil Service Reform Experience," *Review of Public Personnel Administration* 7 (Spring 1987): 72–79; or James D. Slack, "Information, Training, and Assistance Needs of Municipal Governments," *Public Administration Review* 50 (July/August 1990): 450–57.

It was important to assess the methodological utility of combining the various items into the distinctive scales to measure the dependent and independent variables. In other words, it was necessary to determine whether a CAO's response to one item within a particular scale was consistent with his or her responses to the other items within the same scale. To address this concern, Cronbach's alpha was used to test for internal consistency within each of the dependent and independent variable scales.[29] This is a very conservative measure in that the actual reliability of the index can never be lower than the Cronbach's alpha score.[30] Reported in table 16, the Cronbach's alpha scores suggest that each of the scales used shows sufficient levels of internal consistency. Therefore it makes sense to combine the specific items within each scale.

MUNICIPAL GOVERNMENT PREPAREDNESS

How prepared are local governments to manage the workplace ramifications of HIV/AIDS? To answer this question, we must examine the extent to which municipal organizations (1) integrate the ADA into the workplace and (2) make available a variety of HIV/AIDS-related programs and activities. It is first necessary, however, to consider the experience of local government in dealing with HIV/AIDS at the workplace as well as CAO estimates of the prevalence of HIV in the workforce.

Experience with HIV/AIDS and Anticipation

How much experience does local government have in dealing with HIV/AIDS-related situations in its own workforce? In 1989, 7.1 percent of respondents (n = 510) answered yes when asked whether "the city has already had to deal with an HIV/AIDS-related situation in its workforce"; in 1994, the figure was 10.1 percent (n = 507). In short, the figures are small but growing. Between 1989 and 1994, the number of workplace situations involving HIV/AIDS increased by over 40 percent.

When asked to estimate the current number of municipal employees that city managers and mayors believe to be infected with the retrovirus, there is a similar pattern. The overwhelming majority say they believe no employees are infected, but as table 17 shows, the numbers have grown in the last several years. In the late 1980s, CAOs believed that an average of 0.63 city employees had HIV/AIDS. The average drops to 0.18 city employees when the one outlier, the municipality estimating 200 cases of HIV in its workforce, is excluded from consideration. At that time, CAOs in only fourteen municipalities, or approximately 3 percent of the cases, estimated that at least one of their employees was in the HIV spectrum.

Looking at the figures for the mid-1990s, we see that a greater number of CAOs believe that more of their own employees are probably infected with the retrovirus. Today almost 20 percent of local government managers suspect that at least one of their employees has HIV/AIDS; this is an increase of more than 450 percent since the late 1980s. Moreover, CAOs believe that on average each municipality employs 0.71 seropositive workers.

Integrating the ADA into the Workplace

How much do municipal employees know about the ADA? As reported in table 18, almost all local governments provide information about federal antidiscrimination legislation to employees. Slightly less than half, however, have appointed a specialist to handle issues and questions pertaining to HIV/AIDS-related workplace discrimination.[31] Asked whether "the city is prepared to investigate complaints from employees about HIV/AIDS-related discrimination at the workplace," 41.0 percent (n = 519) answered yes in 1989, and 76.3 percent (n = 507) answered yes in 1994.

HIV/AIDS-Related Activities

City managers and mayors were asked whether a specific HIV/AIDS plan had been developed in their respective workplaces. As reported in table 19, more than 15 percent of the CAOs report that they have adopted a set of formal procedures. This number represents a substantial increase since the late 1980s, when nearly nine

Table 17. Estimated Number of HIV/AIDS-Infected Employees in the Municipal Workforce

1989		1994	
Estimate of Cases[a]	Number of Municipalities[b]	Estimate of Cases[c]	Number of Municipalities[d]
0	434	0	335
1	3	1	22
2	3	2	24
3	1	3	13
*	*	4	2
5	1	5	4
6	1	6	2
*	*	8	1
*	*	10	1
*	*	11	1
12	1	*	*
14	1	*	*
15	1	15	1
*	*	20	2
25	2	25	1
*	*	30	1
*	*	35	1
*	*	40	1
*	*	80	1
200	1	*	*

Note: Asterisks indicate that there were no data to report.
[a] Total = 283.   [b] Total = 449.   [c] Total = 295.   [d] Total = 413.

out of ten municipalities in the United States had not yet adopted official guidelines to deal with HIV/AIDS in the workplace.

Municipalities provide different kinds of activities to assist employees with HIV/AIDS and do so in varying degrees. The findings in table 20 suggest three patterns. First, local governments tend to focus efforts on providing technical services and outside referrals much more than they do on providing education and training. Second, the level of HIV/AIDS activities in the mid-1990s has increased substantially since the late 1980s. Third, very few municipalities in the 1980s or the 1990s have experimented with voluntary HIV antibody blood testing procedures in the workplace.

Table 21 reports the level of preparedness in providing reasonable accommoda-

Table 18. Integration of the Americans with Disabilities Act into the
Workplace: Questionnaire Response (percent)

Item	Yes	No
The city provides information to employees about the Americans with Disabilities Act. (n = 507)	86.3	13.7
The city has appointed a specialist to handle all issues pertaining to the Americans with Disabilities Act. (n = 507)	48.9	51.1

Table 19. Municipalities That Adopted an HIV/AIDS Plan for the Workplace,
1989 and 1994 (percent)

Item	Percent
Municipalities in 1989 (n = 522)	10.7
Municipalities in 1994 (n = 505)	15.4

tions to HIV/AIDS employees and job applicants. Two patterns are apparent. First, there seems to be a general commitment to the idea of reasonable accommodations, which is indicated by responses to item 1. Only about half of the CAOs, however, report that they are prepared to provide HIV/AIDS employees with reasonable accommodations of specific sorts, like modifying work schedules, equipment, and training materials. Slightly more than one-third of the city managers and mayors report that they are prepared to modify promotion tests or to provide readers and interpreters for employees with HIV/AIDS, and less than one-third are prepared to pay for necessary reasonable accommodations. This pattern follows the trend in CAO attitudes toward reasonable accommodations that I discussed in Chapter 4: CAOs tend to support the particulars of reasonable accommodation much less than the general concept of reasonable accommodation.

As discussed in Chapter 3, both the Rehab Act and the ADA require city managers and mayors to accommodate job applicants with HIV/AIDS and seropositive employees in similar ways. The second pattern, however, suggests that this is not the case. Across all items in table 21, municipal CAOs show less commitment to the job-related needs of infected applicants than to those of infected employees.

Table 20. HIV/AIDS Workplace Assistance: Practices by Municipalities in the
United States (percent)

Action by the City	1989		1994	
	Yes	n	Yes	n
Is prepared to refer employees concerned about HIV/ AIDS to agencies that offer supportive services	45.3	517	79.9	508
Is prepared to provide HIV/ AIDS employees with benefit consultations to assist them in managing health, leave, and other benefits	22.4	517	62.7	504
Is prepared to provide disability retirement to HIV/AIDS employees when their condition warrants	40.7	518	71.9	469
Provides information about HIV/AIDS to its employees	43.9	522	41.8	507
Provides an HIV/AIDS educa- tion program for its employees	19.9	522	22.6	509
Provides training for supervisors on how to deal with employees with HIV/AIDS	—[a]	—[a]	18.8	504
Has established a voluntary HIV antibody blood testing proce- dure	5.6	519	8.7	506

[a] Item not included in the 1989 survey.

EXPLANATORY FORCES

The impact of background factors on local government preparedness was examined through two statistical procedures: discriminant analysis and multiple regression analysis. The four dependent variables were measured as dichotomous variables. Independent variables either were dichotomous or used interval-level data.
Ordinal and nominal nondichotomous indicators were transposed into dummy variables.

A stepwise multiple regression equation examined the variance in three depen-

Table 21. Level of Preparedness in Making Reasonable Accommodation for
Employees and Job Applicants with HIV/AIDS (percent)

Capacity of the City	For Employees with HIV/AIDS		For Job Applicants with HIV/AIDS	
	Yes	n	Yes	n
Make workplace accommodation similar to those made for people with other disabilities	72.2	500	57.6	507
Modify the work schedules to meet their workplace needs	52.5	499	41.8	500
Restructure jobs to meet their workplace needs	48.9	501	38.4	508
Acquire or modify equipment to meet their workplace needs	52.1	501	50.0	508
To provide qualified readers or interpreters to meet their workplace needs	34.7	493	28.7	501
To modify tests to meet their workplace needs	38.7	489	31.7	489
To modify training materials to meet their workplace needs	56.8	495	52.6	504
Transfer them to other areas if they request such transfers	56.2	498	—[a]	—
Pay for all necessary workplace assistance or accommodation	31.9	495	24.6	504

[a] Not required for compliance with Rehabilitation Act or the Americans with Disabilities Act.

dent variables: adoption of HIV/AIDS workplace assistance practices, reasonable accommodations for employees with HIV/AIDS, and reasonable accommodations for job applicants with HIV/AIDS. Unstandardized regression coefficients, b, measured one-unit change in each independent variable that produced a change in the dependent variable. Standardized regression coefficients, beta, indicated which independent variables best explained the variance in the dependent variable. The larger the absolute value of beta, the stronger the influence of the independent variable. The multiple R statistic indicates the degree of association between the group of independent variables and the dependent variable. By convention, a high level of association would result in a multiple R of ±0.7 to 1.0, and a moderate level of association would produce a multiple R in the range of ±0.3 to 0.7. The coefficient of

Table 22. Determinants of Preparedness: Adopting HIV/AIDS Procedures: Discriminant Analysis

Variable	Unstandardized Coefficient	Standardized Coefficient	Significance F
Personal characteristics			
Unsupportive workplace attitudes	−.58	−.42	.04
Knowledge of HIV/ AIDS	.58	.29	.00
Knowledge of ADA	.62	.30	.00
Organizational environment			
Staff size	.17	.51	.00
Urban setting	.67	.02	.02
Experience with HIV/AIDS			
HIV/AIDS-related situations	1.13	.32	.00

Note: Discriminant analysis eliminated the following indicators due to insufficient levels ($p > .05$) of statistical significance: supportive workplace attitudes, supportive attitudes toward reasonable accommodation, age, race, gender, education, ideology, form of government, population, and estimated number of workers with HIV/AIDS.

determination, R^2, indicates the proportion of the total variation of the dependent variable that is explained by variation in all the independent variables combined.

Because of the nature of the other dependent variable, "HIV/AIDS plans," multiple regression was able to discern little variation. Discriminant analysis, which assesses the utility of independent variables in predicting the classification, or values, of dichotomous, nonscaled dependent variables, was more appropriate. This technique was therefore used to explain why municipalities adopt official HIV/AIDS procedures and policies. The interpretation of its statistics, unstandardized and standardized canonical discriminant function coefficients, is very similar to the b and the beta, respectively, in multiple regression analysis.

Table 22 reports the result of discriminant analysis. A look at the unstandardized coefficients indicates that for every increase in HIV/AIDS-related situations in the workplace, we can expect an increase (1.13) in the likelihood that a municipality will adopt a formal HIV/AIDS policy. To a lesser extent, the same is true in the case of practitioners in urban areas (.67) who have knowledge about the ADA (.62) and about HIV/AIDS (.58) and who do not hold nonsupportive workplace attitudes about HIV/AIDS and the workplace (−.58).

Table 23. Ability of Background Factors to Predict the Adoption of HIV/
AIDS Guidelines (percent)

| | | Predicted Group Membership | | | |
| | | Not Adopted | | Have Adopted | |
Condition	Actual Membership	No.	%	No.	%
Did not adopt HIV/ AIDS guidelines	317	252	79.5	65	20.5
Adopted HIV/AIDS guidelines	53	20	37.7	33	62.3

The standardized coefficients shed additional light on the importance of the independent variables in predicting the adoption of AIDS plans. A higher coefficient means that a given variable has greater power in the discriminant function that is used to predict the values of the dependent variable. We can see that (1) organizations that employ greater numbers of people, (2) CAOs with less unsupportive attitudes toward HIV/AIDS in the workplace, (3) organizations with greater experience dealing with HIV/AIDS-related situations, and (4) CAOs having knowledge about the ADA and an understanding about HIV/AIDS are the most powerful contributors to the discriminant function. That is, these are the best predictors of whether a municipality will (or will not) adopt a formal set of HIV/AIDS policies.

The ability of the independent variables to predict the adoption of HIV/AIDS plans is reported in table 23. Discriminant analysis indicates that all the background factors are able to predict correctly, approximately 80 percent of the time, municipalities that have not adopted HIV/AIDS guidelines. Moreover, the selected independent variables are able to predict municipalities that have adopted HIV/AIDS guidelines slightly more than 60 percent of the time. In other words, our ability to explain why some municipalities have developed HIV/AIDS plans, while others have not, is enhanced considerably by the independent variables comprising the model.

Table 24 reports the effects of the three sets of independent factors on the dependent variable "HIV/AIDS workplace assistance activities." The equation produces moderate levels (multiple $R = .56$) of association. The adjusted R^2 value indicates that the equation explains 32 percent of the variance in whether or not a municipal government provides HIV/AIDS workplace assistance activities. The multiple R and R^2 values are substantial, given that large numbers of variables in a regression model often deflate the true influence of the regression statistics.

Analysis of the unstandardized regression coefficients in table 24 suggests that

Table 24. Determinants of Preparedness: HIV/AIDS Workplace Assistance
Activities

Variable	b	Standard Error	Beta	Significance T
Personal characteristics				
Gender (male)	−.75	.30	−.13	.01
Race (Anglo)	1.25	.61	.10	.04
College education				
(graduate-level)	.46	.23	.10	.05
Knowledge of ADA	1.22	.23	.26	.00
Belief that HIV/AIDS				
plan is needed	.84	.23	.17	.00
Supportive workplace				
attitudes	.43	.61	.22	.00
Organizational environment				
Staff size	.00	4.50	.14	.02
Experience with HIV/AIDS				
HIV/AIDS-related				
situations	1.33	.46	.16	.01
Constant	4.23	1.52	—	—

Note: Multiple R = .56. Standard error = 1.96. Adjusted R^2 = .32. Significance $F \leq .00$. Discriminant analysis eliminated the following indicators because of insufficient levels ($p > .05$) of statistical significance: nonsupportive workplace attitudes, supportive attitudes toward reasonable accommodation, age, ideology, form of government, and estimated number of workers with HIV/AIDS.

three factors are important in changing the level of preparedness. Experience with HIV/AIDS-related situations ($b = 1.33$), CAOs' whiteness ($b = 1.25$), and knowledge about the ADA ($b = 1.22$) tend to increase the chances that municipal governments will provide HIV/AIDS assistance activities. For example, for every one-unit change in the extent to which organizations gain experience in dealing with HIV/AIDS-related situations, there is a 1.33 unit change in providing assistance. To a lesser extent, the belief that an HIV/AIDS plan is needed, and the presence of a female CAO, also mean a change in whether or not a city provides assistance activities.

Analysis of the standardized regression coefficients indicates that two factors— knowledge about the ADA (beta = .26) and supportive workplace attitudes (beta = .22)—together have the greatest explanatory power in determining the variance in level of assistance activities. That is, these factors are best for predicting whether or

Table 25. Determinants of Preparedness: Reasonable Accommodation for
Employees with HIV/AIDS

Variable	b	Standard Error	Beta	Significance T
Personal characteristics				
Gender (male)	1.04	.36	.13	.00
Age	−.05	.01	−.15	.00
Race (Anglo)	1.70	.75	.10	.02
College education (graduate-level)	.73	.29	.11	.01
Supportive attitudes toward reasonable accommodation	.70	.15	.22	.00
Belief that HIV/AIDS plan is needed	.66	.26	.10	.02
Supportive workplace attitudes	.81	.14	.30	.00
Nonsupportive workplace attitudes	−.49	.21	−.12	.02
Organizational environment				
Staff size	.00	4.63	.14	.00
Experience with HIV/AIDS	—	—	—	—
Constant	4.23	1.52	—	—

Note: Multiple R = .67. Standard error = 2.40. Adjusted R^2 = .43 Significance F ≤ .00. Discriminant analysis eliminated the following indicators because of insufficient levels (p > .05) of statistical significance: ideology, knowledge about ADA, knowledge about HIV/AIDS, form of government, community setting, citizens opposed to hiring HIV/AIDS individuals, estimated number of workers with HIV/AIDS, experience with HIV/AIDS situations, council expressed concern over hiring HIV/AIDS individuals.

not a municipal government provides these activities. To a lesser extent, believing that an HIV/AIDS plan is needed (beta = .17) and having experience dealing with HIV/AIDS-related situations (beta = .16) also have predictive value.

Table 25 reports the results of regressing the third dependent variable, "providing reasonable accommodation for employees with HIV/AIDS," onto the three clusters of independent variables. This regression equation produces a moderate level of association (multiple R = .67) and the adjusted R^2 value indicates that the independent variables explain over 43 percent of the variance in providing reasonable accommodations to employees with HIV/AIDS.

Analysis of the unstandardized regression coefficients suggests that two factors are important in changing the level of reasonable accommodations provided to employees with HIV/AIDS: CAOs' whiteness ($b = 1.70$) and maleness ($b = 1.04$). To a lesser extent, other factors produce changes in this dimension of preparedness: graduate-level education ($b = .73$), supportive workplace attitudes ($b = .81$), supportive attitudes toward reasonable accommodation ($b = .70$), and a belief that an HIV/AIDS plan is needed ($b = .66$). The standardized regression coefficients confirm the importance of CAO attitudes in explaining the variance, especially those that center on the person with HIV/AIDS in the work setting (beta = .30) and the employee's right to access reasonable accommodations (beta = .22). Other factors, such as the youthfulness of CAOs (beta = −.15) and larger organizational size (beta = .14), also have some explanatory value.

Table 26 shows the statistical results involving the fourth and final dependent variable, "providing reasonable accommodation for HIV/AIDS job applicants." This equation also produces a moderate level of association (multiple $R = .67$). The adjusted R^2 indicates that the regression model explains 45 percent of the variance.

The unstandardized regression coefficients indicate that several factors produce changes in the level of preparedness to provide reasonable accommodations to job applicants with HIV/AIDS: male CAOs ($b = .98$), supportive workplace attitudes ($b = .81$), and the perception that citizens are *not* opposed to the hiring of people with HIV/AIDS ($b = −.74$). To a lesser extent, supportive attitudes toward reasonable accommodation ($b = .63$), the belief that an HIV/AIDS plan is needed ($b = .62$), and graduate-level education ($b = .57$) also produce changes in the dependent variable. The standardized regression coefficients suggest that two variables, supportive workplace attitudes (beta = .34) and supportive attitudes toward reasonable accommodations (beta = .22), provide the best predictive power in determining whether or not a municipal government is prepared to provide reasonable accommodations to job applicants.

CONCLUSIONS

While there has been improvement since the late 1980s, local governments remain ill prepared to manage most of the workplace ramifications of the HIV/AIDS epidemic. More municipalities have experience in dealing with HIV/AIDS situations, and more city managers and mayors provide higher estimates of the probability of HIV prevalence within their respective workforces. Yet it is also quite possible that the proportion of seropositive employees is nearly three times greater than practitioners suspect.[32] Overwhelmingly, local governments also provide information about the ADA to their employees, and compared with the late 1980s, many more are prepared to investigate complaints about HIV/AIDS-related discrimination.

More city halls have adopted formal sets of procedures to deal with HIV/AIDS in the workplace than did so in the late 1980s, but the number is still disturb-

Table 26. Determinants of Preparedness: Reasonable Accommodation for Job
Applicants with HIV/AIDS

Variable	b	Standard Error	Beta	Significance T
Personal characteristics				
Gender (male)	.98	.32	.14	.00
Age	−.05	.01	−.16	.00
College education				
(graduate-level)	.57	.26	.14	.03
Supportive attitudes				
toward reasonable				
accommodation	.63	.13	.22	.00
Belief that HIV/AIDS				
plan is needed	.62	.26	.10	.02
Supportive workplace				
attitudes	.81	.11	.34	.00
Organizational environment				
Staff size	.00	4.17	.14	.00
Citizens opposed to				
hiring HIV/AIDS				
individuals	−.74	.26	−.12	.00
Experience with HIV/AIDS	—	—	—	—
Constant	4.31	1.32	—	—

Note: Multiple R = .67. Standard error = 2.16. Adjusted R^2 = .45. Significance $F \leq$ .00. Discriminant analysis eliminated the following indicators because of insufficient levels ($p > .05$) of statistical significance: race, ideology, knowledge about ADA, knowledge about HIV/AIDS, nonsupportive attitudes, form of government, community setting, estimated number of workers with HIV/AIDS, experience with HIV/AIDS situations, council expressed concern over hiring HIV/AIDS individuals.

ingly small. Similarly, more local governments provide an array of disparate HIV/ AIDS-related activities, but efforts still vary in level and type. The trend seems to be to offer activities that are more reactive (e.g., referrals to outside organizations and benefit consultation) than proactive (e.g., employee education and training). From the perspective of the CAO, activities chosen are probably viewed as being strategies of least expense. In part from a concern about cost, the limited consensus on the issue of reasonable accommodation declines further when the discussion shifts from abstract concepts to concrete options. Furthermore, there is much less support for providing reasonable accommodations for job applicants with HIV/ AIDS than for providing reasonable accommodations for current employees with HIV/AIDS.

Does the organization's experience with HIV/AIDS make a difference in the level of preparedness? Its greatest impact seems to be in determining when a municipality adopts an HIV/AIDS plan and, to a lesser extent, the level of disparate activities it offers. But experience with HIV/AIDS seems to have little bearing on decisions regarding reasonable accommodations.

Does the organization's environment make a difference? While the size of the workforce affects the level of preparedness, most other factors do not. The fact that a municipality is located in an urban area has only a slight impact on the adoption of formal HIV/AIDS plans. Neither the size of the community nor the form of government has any effect. Organizations run by big-city mayors are as poorly prepared as those administered by small-town professional managers.

Personal attributes of CAOs can play an important role in the group dynamics needed to build greater responsive capacity within organizations, but how great an influence they exert depends on the background characteristics examined. Contrary to politically correct thinking, for instance, one's ideology has little impact on the level and quality of responsiveness. Liberal CAOs are just as poorly prepared to manage HIV/AIDS situations as their more conservative counterparts.

Other factors seem to make a difference. Younger and more educated CAOs may be much more in tune with the complex issues of the day—both inside the work setting and outside it. That race and gender, especially whiteness and maleness, can also make positive contributions should come as no surprise. Public servants with either attribute may be learning to play the role of "active representative" more effectively and may therefore be adding an important factor into the workplace diversity equation.[33] That white males are sensitive on the issue of HIV/AIDS may also be the much-sought-after product of fundamental changes that have been implemented in higher education during the last decade or so.[34]

More than demographic attributes, however, the opinions and views of individuals can play an important role in building a supportive workplace environment and in meeting the needs of employees and job applicants with HIV/AIDS. Particularly important are knowledge about federal legislation and enlightened and legally informed views about the workplace ramifications of the retrovirus. The findings here suggest that CAO attitudes, regardless of the particular personnel background characteristics, can go a long way in changing the organizational culture in relation to HIV/AIDS.

A substantial number of city governments (more than in the late 1980s) are today approaching step 2 in the emergency management process: they are developing responsive strategies for dealing with the workplace ramifications of HIV/AIDS.[35] A few more municipalities have entered steps 3 and 4 of the emergency management process: they are actually assisting members of the workforce who are in the HIV spectrum and are trying to restore the workplace to normalcy. But the vast majority of municipalities appear to fall somewhere between step 1 (deciding what to do) and step 2, and as in the late 1980s, many continue to be so unprepared that they are not even at step 1.

The findings have a direct bearing on the dynamics of the public service from at least three vantage points. First, the plight of seropositive workers is exacerbated by insufficient levels of preparation. In Chapter 4, I argued that, as a result of practitioners' mixed attitudes, employees in the HIV spectrum may feel the need to choose between advocating for their own workplace rights and remaining silent about their condition from fear of discrimination. The absence of enough institutionalized support mechanisms, in the form of plans and practices, also underscores the perception of inconsistency and uncertainty in the workplace environment.

Consequently, seropositive employees might decide to delay, for as long as possible, reporting their health conditions and needs for reasonable accommodation to either supervisors or personnel specialists. Low estimates of seropositive individuals in the workforce, as well as the low proportion of city governments with experience in HIV/AIDS-related situations, may be evidence that they are doing so. It might simply be easier for someone dying of AIDS to hide his or her symptoms and not expend energy "fighting city hall," even though that decision would mean that the person would not receive desperately needed assistance and benefits. If this is the case for employees with HIV/AIDS, it is certainly true for job applicants with HIV/AIDS.

Second, the low levels of preparedness shed light on the nature of HIV/AIDS decision making in local government. As in the late 1980s, city managers and mayors continue to take a cautious and reactive approach to managing this crisis, as shown by the statistics. More Americans have contracted AIDS than died on both sides of the American Civil War, making the HIV/AIDS epidemic the worst disaster in American history. And yet fewer than two out of ten municipalities in the United States have adopted an HIV/AIDS plan. Although on average more than two members of every local government workforce are probably seropositive, approximately eight out of ten municipalities still have not established either HIV/AIDS education programs for all employees or HIV/AIDS training programs for supervisory staff.

City managers and mayors respond to HIV/AIDS in the workplace only when the need to do so is undeniable. The fact that practitioners underestimate the number of seropositive workers simply reinforces this process; nothing is done if HIV/AIDS is not perceived as a problem. We should therefore remember that, while the organization's memory affects the current level of preparedness, it does so without regard to the inaccuracy of information it absorbs.

In addition, local government decision making about HIV/AIDS is characterized by incrementalism. And this characteristic lends credence to the uncertainty expressed by practitioners in Chapter 4. Perhaps because they want to do what is right for all within the community, they strive for a balance between doing nothing about a very real crisis and overreacting to what may appear to be an extremely limited situation. The process seems to take the following pattern.

City governments with no known workers in the HIV spectrum do nothing about HIV/AIDS. Those with a few seropositive employees may develop some disparate HIV/AIDS assistance activities, ranging from providing information about the disease to making various kinds of reasonable accommodations. As the number of HIV cases grows, the need for a more pronounced and systematic response becomes increasingly evident and eventually culminates in the adoption of formal HIV/AIDS plans.

This interpretation explains why the size of the municipal staff has the highest predictive value (table 22, beta = .51, where beta is the standardized coefficient) in determining the adoption of an HIV/AIDS plan. It also explains why changes in the urbanness of the environment (table 22, b = .67, where b is the unstandardized coefficient) alter the chances of adopting such a plan. Local governments in larger and urban settings have had to go further in their preparations for dealing with the workplace ramifications of HIV/AIDS because they have a greater need to respond to actual situations involving the retrovirus (table 22, b = 1.13, beta = .32). City managers and mayors in larger and more urban municipalities have had more time and reason to develop and adopt formal HIV/AIDS plans than their counterparts in smaller and less urban municipalities.

The fact that governments make decisions lethargically and incrementally should come as no surprise. They typically respond to all types of problems in this manner. After all, government faces many daily crises, and one of the central tasks of the practitioner is to refrain from expending more human and material resources than are really needed to address a particular problem at a particular moment. But the fact is that cities cannot address the needs of seropositive employees and job applicants in the same way that they fill in potholes, buy snow removal equipment, or fund recreation programs. Routine decision making, which may be sufficient in other policy matters, becomes terribly inappropriate in managing the HIV/AIDS crisis because it hinders planning and preparedness.

The third implication centers on the capacity of local government to deliver services to the community. Preparedness is partially a function of the access that city managers and mayors have to HIV/AIDS-related education and training opportunities. These activities will certainly add to the cost of running the internal side of bureaucracy. Practitioners' underestimates of the number of seropositive employees suggest that local government cannot escape being faced with workplace-related costs for HIV/AIDS that will be more than two times greater than is currently feared.[36] The fact that adequate support mechanisms are not in place only exacerbates the situation, because individuals in the HIV spectrum are productive for longer periods of time when they receive treatment and reasonable accommodations while the retrovirus is still in its earliest stages. When seropositive workers and job applicants conceal their condition, the cost to the local government organization increases in terms of more expensive medical treatments and more frequent training of new, replacement personnel.

Given that the costs of supervisory and personnel training, health care benefits, and providing reasonable accommodation are lower today than they will be tomorrow, tough choices will have to be made about the quality of services delivered in every community. Which programs will continue to receive scarce and limited tax dollars? Which ones are destined for either cutbacks or termination? While such decisions cannot be avoided, they can be made more rationally and efficiently if local government increases planning and preparedness in addressing the HIV/AIDS crisis in the workplace.

6

HIV/AIDS and the Public Service
The Crisis Revisited

THE CRISIS that the HIV/AIDS epidemic is creating in the public service has the potential to alter fundamental relationships between people and their governments. From the citizen's perspective, the crisis can best be seen and felt on the external side of bureaucracy. HIV/AIDS increasingly affects the quality of services available as well as the manner in which those services are delivered.

The crisis has its genesis, however, in the internal side of bureaucracy. Decisions about the type of people hired, the nature of their jobs, and the nature of the organizational environment ultimately determine the amount of additional funding that will be needed to replenish personnel line items, fringe benefits, health care coverage, and general operating budgets.

The effects of the crisis on both sides of bureaucracy are interactive. In these times when the public service is faced with limited revenues, the eras of so-called cutback management and government reinvention, the reallocation of resources to cover these expenses exacerbates the effects of the retrovirus on the quality and manner of service delivery.

This book has focused on the HIV/AIDS epidemic from the standpoint of the internal side of bureaucracy in local governments. A public emergency management standard was applied in that local government preparedness was operationalized by having either a comprehensive plan or at least some activities in place to address the workplace ramifications of HIV/AIDS. Four central concerns have been raised about HIV/AIDS and the workforce. First, how prepared is local government? Second, can practitioners screen job applicants and current employees to determine who is in the HIV spectrum? Third, where does the balance lie between the worker's right to confidentiality on health matters and the citizen's right to know about issues that may affect service delivery and the tax base? Fourth, what is the appropriate relationship between public employees within the HIV spectrum and the citizenry? Answers to these questions are found not only in epidemiological and legal expectations but also in the discretion exercised by practitioners in making personnel decisions and shaping the workplace environment.

FINDINGS

How prepared are local governments to manage the workplace ramifications of this epidemic? As we have seen, most are not, perhaps because they believe that the epidemic has not yet reached their communities. While a majority of city managers and mayors are now prepared to investigate HIV/AIDS-related workplace discrimination, few are cognizant of the legal rights of employees and job applicants in the HIV spectrum when it comes to providing reasonable accommodations. Fewer than one in five have developed HIV/AIDS guidelines for the workplace, although the number of organizations with such plans has increased since the late 1980s. In 1994, compared with the late 1980s, more city managers and mayors have instituted HIV/AIDS-related practices, but few have developed education and training programs as yet.

Practitioners may screen job applicants and current employees to determine who is in the HIV spectrum only in specific situations. The Rehab Act and the ADA permit such screening after an offer is made to a job applicant and then only if the screening is (1) narrowly focused, (2) job related, (3) consistent with business necessity, and (4) applied to all personnel within a particular job classification. Some areas of local government, especially in the public safety and emergency-response fields, may qualify for the utilization of HIV antibody blood testing as a postemployment screening device.

Where does the balance lie between the worker's right to confidentiality on health matters and the citizen's right to know about issues that may impact service delivery and the tax base? The courts have ruled that the employee's right to privacy about health issues far outweighs all other concerns of the citizenry. The issue of reasonable accommodation, however, makes it much more difficult to maintain the traditional view of confidentiality in the workplace. More people within the organization will need to know something about a person's disability if that organization chooses to provide *effective* accommodations, rather than simply reasonable accommodations, and thereby seeks to observe the spirit as well as the letter of the law.

Since the courts have determined that seropositive public servants do not necessarily present a danger to others, the appropriate relationship between them and the public is predicated on the general rules that govern safe and healthy interactions among everyone. A local government employee who is bleeding should have contact with neither citizen nor coworker, regardless of the HIV status of the people involved. Epidemiological common sense also suggests that a seropositive employee should probably refrain from close contact with people who are ill, regardless of whether they are citizens or coworkers.

A notable proportion of city managers and mayors do express concerns on key issues that run contrary to legal expectations. For instance, they continue to be uncertain on the issue of HIV antibody blood testing as a screening device;

many would like to see it used more broadly in the workplace. In the mid-1990s as throughout the history of the HIV/AIDS epidemic, local government practitioners remain concerned about the epidemiological and political ramifications of permitting direct contact between the citizenry and employees in the HIV spectrum. Many practitioners are also torn between maintaining the confidentiality of the employee's health condition and acknowledging the right of citizens to know about the workings of government and to have information about individuals who are employed by city hall.

In essence, the fish bowl environment of the public sector affects the way practitioners view HIV/AIDS. In the late 1980s one local government official remarked, "Unfortunately, the same standards of conduct do not exist in the public sector as they do in the private sector. Public employees are very limited on what is personal and a matter of public record. That may not be their perception—but it is the reality." The same seems to be true in the mid-1990s.

What forces affect local government preparedness? The model used in this study, with nearly 65 percent certainty, predicts factors that lead to the adoption of formal HIV/AIDS plans in municipalities throughout the nation. With nearly 80 percent certainty, it also predicts the factors that *do not* lead to the adoption of formal HIV/AIDS plans. In addition to the size of the city's workforce and organizational experience in dealing with HIV/AIDS-related situations, the factors with apparently the greatest effect on HIV/AIDS plan adoptions center on the personal characteristics of the CAO: workplace attitudes toward people with HIV/AIDS, knowledge of the law, and knowledge of HIV/AIDS.

The model also explains nearly one-third of the variance in local government's decision to provide HIV/AIDS-related assistance activities in the workplace. The city hall most likely to have disparate policies and programs on line is one that has a large workforce and experience dealing with HIV/AIDS-related situations. As in the case of the adoption of formal plans, personal characteristics of the city manager or mayor make it easier to implement HIV/AIDS-related assistance activities: knowledge of the laws and the belief that an HIV/AIDS plan is needed. It is also helpful if the CAO is a white woman with a graduate-level degree.

In addition, the model explains approximately 45 percent of the variance in local government preparedness with respect to providing reasonable accommodations to job applicants and employees with HIV/AIDS. Personal attributes of CAOs overwhelmingly influence the availability of reasonable accommodations for employees with HIV/AIDS. Local governments are most prepared when the CAO is a younger white male with graduate-level education, has positive attitudes regarding both the workplace and reasonable accommodation, and believes in the need for an HIV/AIDS plan. Except for race, similar personal factors affect the preparedness of local government to provide reasonable accommodations to job applicants with HIV/AIDS. But here the anticipation of citizen reaction also plays an important role. The experience of an organization in dealing with HIV/AIDS-related situations, however, has no impact on local government preparedness in providing reasonable accommodations to either job applicant or employee in the HIV spectrum.

IMPLICATIONS

Implications for the public service are three. First, the work environment in the 1990s is filled with uncertainty and ambiguity. City managers and mayors typically do not know what to do in the case of HIV/AIDS, and support mechanisms are not always in place. As a result, seropositive workers and job applicants cannot always be sure about what will happen if they disclose their condition to supervisors or interviewers. Will reasonable accommodations be provided? Will they be treated with respect and understanding? Will they be ostracized or even discharged for erroneous reasons? These very real fears may lead many employees and job applicants in the HIV spectrum to remain silent.

Second, the findings show that local governments are slow in responding to the HIV/AIDS crisis in the workplace. They react piecemeal and only when there is clear evidence that the epidemic has reached their workforce. Because the vast majority of local governments are not preparing in advance, they typically lack the requisite information, training, and resources prior to the first HIV/AIDS case. As a result, practitioners may be unable to manage the crisis in an effective, humane, and legal manner.

Third, the cost of HIV/AIDS to local government will be much greater than necessary. As discussed in Chapter 2, the workplace cost for each seropositive employee with an annual salary of $25,000 will range from about $135,000 in municipalities with group health care packages to about $210,000 in self-insured municipalities. These costs are assumed to cover a thirteen-year period. Because of local government's underestimation of the number of HIV-positive workers, the costs may be double that which is anticipated for the entire workforce. In addition, drug therapies using protease inhibitors may extend the length and quality of life for many seropositive people and thereby raise the workplace cost of the epidemic even more.

Moreover, these estimates assume a responsive, and even proactive, workplace, one with a supportive environment that provides early intervention in the form of varied assistance activities and reasonable accommodations. The findings here, however, suggest that the local government workplace is not very responsive and proactive. When seropositive workers and job applicants delay disclosing their health conditions, they tend to become less productive and actually deplete sick days and health care benefit packages at a faster rate than if they had begun treatment during earlier stages of the retrovirus. The ultimate cost of burying and replacing personnel will accrue much more quickly in this kind of environment.

But the greatest expense for the unprepared workplace will be in the area of

litigation. While currently only a small proportion of ADA-based workplace litigation stems from HIV/AIDS-related situations, the number of lawsuits is growing as
managers begin to respond to an increasing number of requests for reasonable accommodations.[1] We can expect litigation involving local government and individuals requesting reasonable accommodation to be particularly keen, given both the
attitudes of CAOs and the low levels of preparedness to provide such assistance in
their respective workplaces. The findings suggest that the largest number of lawsuits
might stem from the "otherwise qualified" seropositive job applicant who seeks reasonable accommodations to allow him or her the opportunity to perform the essential functions of the advertised position. Given the limited revenue sources in most
communities, local governments may have to reduce or curtail some public services
in order to meet the additional internal expenses resulting from HIV/AIDS.

WHY ARE LOCAL GOVERNMENTS UNPREPARED?

All evidence suggests that the HIV/AIDS epidemic will be one of the worst
disasters to strike the United States. More Americans died of AIDS in 1992, for instance, than died as a result of combat during our entire eight-year involvement
in the Vietnam War.[2] Although protease inhibitors have dramatically lowered the
number of deaths to AIDS, the current number of Americans who have acquired
full-blown AIDS is greater than the number of Americans who died in the Second
World War.[3] As noted earlier, more Americans have full-blown AIDS than died
from involvement in the American Civil War, the most deadly crisis in our history.[4]
The epidemic affects every city and town in every urban and rural setting in every
territory and state. It affects all races and both genders, and over 98 percent of its
victims are of working age. No one is immune, and millions of Americans probably
carry the retrovirus without their knowledge.

Under these circumstances, the most important question seems to be: why do
local governments, the largest source of employment in the United States, remain so
ill prepared to address the workplace ramifications of this epidemic? The easiest
answer, of course, is that most local governments remain unprepared because they
lack the factors that are correlated with having HIV/AIDS plans, assistance activities, and reasonable accommodations in place. More complex reasons have to do
with reliance on the public health model to solve workplace problems and a general
lack of national leadership.

First, the traditional public health model is proving to be an ineffective and inappropriate approach for managing workplace ramifications of HIV/AIDS. Its
hallmark procedures—the dissemination of preventive information, the testing of
at-risk individuals, and epidemiological research—have helped combat the social effects of a wide variety of contagious diseases throughout this century. But the model
provides the employer with neither guidance nor incentives for making internal
workplace decisions.

By relying primarily on the dissemination of preventive information about HIV/AIDS and hoping for a cure, workplace managers shift professional responsibility to public health authorities. Like other employers, city managers and mayors want to believe that the impact of the retrovirus on their workforces will be minimized if public health officials and medical researchers do their jobs properly. The public health model, therefore, affects workplace managers in two ways. First, it enables CAOs to distance themselves from the need to make critical decisions in advance and allows them to adopt more reactive and incremental solutions when they are confronted with an HIV/AIDS-related situation in the workplace. The public health model thus fails to empower workplace managers—and empowerment is essential for compliance with both the letter and the spirit of federal antidiscrimination legislation.

Second, the distancing of the CAO and other workplace supervisors allows political considerations to overshadow legal expectations. The electorate need not act rationally and may very well oust a city manager or mayor who chooses to ignore its concerns in favor of compliance with the law. Such concern about popular support may very well underlie practitioners' rather mixed attitudes toward seropositive employees, reasonable accommodations, HIV antibody testing, and citizen contact. The public health model affords CAOs opportunities to avoid taking positions that may be epidemiologically and legally correct but politically unpopular. In doing so, the approach helps sustain an organizational environment characterized by uncertainty, anxiety, and fear.

The second reason for local government's unpreparedness is the continuing lack of national leadership and direction in managing the HIV/AIDS crisis. Strangely, such leadership is not lacking with other types of public emergencies. When natural or technological disasters occur, for instance, public administrators can rely on the Federal Emergency Management Agency (FEMA) to initiate technical and financial assistance during the response and recovery stages. FEMA can also be instrumental in the preparation and planning phases, by showing what needs to be done and by providing leadership in securing all necessary agreements and coordinating responding agencies.

Many nonprofit and public agencies, like the American Red Cross and the U.S. Centers for Disease Control and Prevention, are available to assist city managers and mayors in coping with the HIV/AIDS epidemic. From Bakersfield to Boston, local AIDS foundations exist to provide some assistance. But these organizations adhere to the public health model and function more as information and data providers than as primary responders to organizational problems incurred as a result of the emergency.

In line with my recommendation in the first edition of this book, the Clinton administration created the position of national AIDS coordinator, or "AIDS czar," which oversees the White House's National AIDS Policy Office. The mission of the National AIDS Policy Office, which was established in 1993, is to coordinate all the activities in the fight against HIV/AIDS and to develop clear policy goals for the White House. Regrettably, the past and current AIDS czars Kristine Gebbie and Patsy Fleming, have not been given the necessary resources and authority to perform the tasks of coordination and direction.[5] The staff of twelve full-time employees can provide little direct assistance to inquiries about HIV/AIDS and the workplace.[6]

The federal government continues to play only a marginal role in addressing HIV/AIDS-related issues in the workplace.[7] Through legislation and court decisions, it regulates behavior but does not distribute resources that might lead to greater levels of preparedness. No single centralized agency assists local governments and other work organizations in coordinating their efforts or in answering the many questions about HIV/AIDS in the workplace. In establishing HIV/AIDS guidelines and assistance activities, city managers and mayors must take on the responsibility of finding outside expertise and perhaps reinventing wheels that are already in place in other work settings. The federal government, moreover, offers no assistance to local government practitioners or other workplace managers in sustaining current ceilings on the cost of health care packages or in financing reasonable accommodations to meet the special workplace needs of seropositive workers. In a very fundamental way, the federal government continues to ignore the daily concerns and needs of all workplace managers, including city managers and mayors, in their efforts to cope effectively with the organizational problems associated with HIV/AIDS.

INCREASING LOCAL GOVERNMENT PREPAREDNESS

Knowing why local government is unprepared to deal with HIV/AIDS is not the same as knowing how to improve its level of preparedness. While the former requires analysis of the past, the latter calls for foresight. Such endeavors can be undertaken in only a tentative fashion. After all, the HIV/AIDS epidemic has underscored the uncertainty of science, and the policy and organizational sciences remain its most imprecise and preparadigmatic siblings. In most instances, we are faced with matters of correlation, not causation. Given the gravity of HIV/AIDS, however, we have no choice but to try to delineate the factors that might improve management's ability to deal with workplace ramifications of the epidemic.

What can be done to increase the level of local government preparedness? This study's findings provide some insights, although not all of the factors are applicable to every community. Small organizations cannot simply become large ones, and the extent of HIV/AIDS-related experience cannot be controlled. But some of the forces with a bearing on the level of preparedness can be manipulated. Given the statistical importance of legal and epidemiological knowledge, for instance, we can search for more effective ways to enlighten practitioners about these issues. We can also attempt to modify and inform employers' opinions about seropositive individuals in the workforce. We can even propose curriculum revisions in order to strengthen the relationship between local government preparedness and graduate-level education. By focusing on those forces that can be altered through individual and organizational efforts, we begin to move away from the reactive-incremental approach toward a more proactive posture.

One way to facilitate this transition is by adopting an emergency management perspective.[8] As discussed throughout this book, the emergency management paradigm has four components: (1) deciding what must be done in the workplace (e.g., what HIV/AIDS-related assistance should be available and what reasonable accommodations should be provided); (2) developing a plan to accomplish necessary tasks (e.g., allocating sufficient funding, designating staff and units responsible for providing specific activities, and disseminating information about the response plan); (3) actually responding to the crisis (e.g., assisting seropositive workers according to the plan of action); and (4) providing support during the period of "recovery" (in the case of HIV/AIDS, striving for an acceptable quality of work life between the time of diagnosis and the time of death). An emergency management approach therefore requires a shift in the primary burden of responsibility for preparedness and action from extraorganizational authorities like public health officials to leadership within the city hall workplace.

Yet it is not an easy task to apply emergency management principles to the HIV/AIDS crisis in the workplace. As discussed in Chapter 2, this retrovirus represents a completely new kind of public emergency. It is one with which we have very limited experience and consequently very little understanding about the appropriate application of management skills. As we have seen, although we know demographically where HIV is currently striking, we cannot pinpoint when it has actually struck. Because we do not fully understand the dynamics of this crisis, it is much harder for us to engage in responsive activities. What we currently lack is the knowledge of how to translate emergency management expertise into concrete actions that assist local government practitioners in confronting this particular crisis more effectively.

Two broad initiatives are in order. First, management must empower itself and accept primary responsibility for finding solutions to the workplace ramifications of HIV/AIDS. Given the stigma associated with the retrovirus, and the Rosa Parks dilemma previously discussed, the quickest way to facilitate the self-empowerment of seropositive workers is for management to take a more proactive stance. If management chooses, it can develop a positive and supportive work environment, one that encourages seropositive employees to seek out necessary job-related assistance that will enable them to remain healthy and productive for the longest period of time. Hence it is in the best interest of the organization, as well as of employees with HIV/AIDS, to develop such an environment. Since the dictates of profit and productivity coincide with the ideal of compassion, managers have every reason to empower themselves and find localized solutions to this complex workplace crisis.

Second, because the HIV/AIDS epidemic presents a national emergency affecting the health, civil rights, and productivity of a growing number of Americans in every location, we simply cannot afford further delays. Management must be encouraged to become proactive, regardless of whether the workplace is in Mississippi or Massachusetts. And even though the current political climate entails reinventing government by downsizing its workforce and contracting out its responsibilities, in this crisis we must access the full regulatory, distributive, and coordinative resources of the federal government.

I am calling for neither liberal nor big government solutions; such labels belong to a brand of politics that has been as problematic in the fight against HIV/AIDS as the politics of conservatism and New Federalism. We should recognize that the use of federal resources for the HIV/AIDS effort fits well within the fashionable tenets of government decentralization and community-based problem solving. Assertive government actions are intended to foster the critical processes of entrepreneurial search and experimentation—prerequisites for securing managerial empowerment and for finding workable solutions within individual workplaces. I am calling for good government, not necessarily Republican or Democratic government, for the use of public resources to develop more proactive local strategies to combat a crisis that affects all Americans.

RECOMMENDATION 1: SELF-EMPOWERMENT OF MANAGEMENT

If we are to increase the level of local government preparedness in dealing with the HIV/AIDS epidemic, CAOs must take control of the situation. In order to maintain a productive workforce, as well as a cost-efficient and compassionate workplace, they must take proactive steps in at least three areas: (1) developing and implementing an HIV/AIDS plan for the workplace, (2) adopting an effective HIV/AIDS training program, and (3) incorporating routine HIV antibody blood testing and counseling into the health practices of the organization and the workforce.

HIV/AIDS Plans for the Workplace

An HIV/AIDS plan can help management accomplish extremely interrelated tasks: minimizing workplace costs and maximizing workers' health, morale, and productivity. First, a formal plan can help management comply with the requirements of both the Rehab Act and the ADA. Issues of confidentiality and reasonable accommodation, for instance, can be incorporated into the language of the plan. In essence, a formal plan can act as a reminder of both the rights of the employee and the obligations of the employer.

Second, an HIV/AIDS plan can help create a positive workplace environment, one that facilitates the self-empowerment of seropositive job applicants and employees. It can help minimize the adverse effects of the Rosa Parks dilemma. Like an equal employment opportunity policy, an HIV/AIDS plan helps set the tone within the organization. It helps both supervisors and employees by defining appropriate conduct and indicating what procedures and services are available. Its acceptance can transform a reactive and hostile workplace into one that fosters proactivity and compassion. Adoption of a formal plan is the first step in building the necessary level of trust between seropositive individuals and management.

Third, an HIV/AIDS plan can also help management control workplace-related costs of HIV/AIDS and maintain current levels of productivity. While an effective plan cannot eliminate costs, it can help managers use materials and human resources more wisely and productively. Knowing how to provide reasonable accommodation, for instance, can postpone and soften the use of health care packages and can delay the costly investment in replacing personnel. Having an HIV/AIDS plan in operation is evidence of intent to provide reasonable accommodations and will therefore help minimize the cost of any litigation incurred when the organization is forced to claim undue hardship. Knowing how to manage the fears and prejudices of coworkers and managers will also help limit the omnipresent threat of lawsuit.

There are currently at least two examples of model plans to deal with the workplace ramifications of HIV/AIDS.[9] In the first edition of this book, a four-part workplace plan was proposed and subsequently enhanced.[10]

The first part of the plan reaffirms management's commitment to implementing the nondiscriminatory principles found within the Rehab Act and the ADA. It is a declaration that the organization supports the workplace rights of seropositive individuals. The second component is designed to protect the employer from lawsuits. It should remind supervisors of the need to maintain strict confidentiality in dealing with employee health matters. This section should also address the fears and possible actions of coworkers.

In the third component of an HIV/AIDS plan, management affirms its commitment to providing reasonable accommodations to HIV positive workers and job applicants. The ADA and the Rehab Act permit discretion in defining reasonable accommodations so that the nature of the work site and the resources of the organization can be taken into account. Management should specify which services and accommodations are available within each specific work site as well as the services available within the community.

The fourth component of the plan is education and training. Education is instrumental in managing the workplace ramifications of HIV/AIDS. Managers and supervisors should receive ongoing training to keep them informed about pertinent litigation and changes in workplace practices relating to HIV/AIDS employees. Workers should receive information that dispels fears about HIV infection at the workplace as well as directives that outline the behavior expected of all employees.

Although the overwhelming majority of local governments still have not developed formal HIV/AIDS plans, some municipalities have done so, and selected documents are compiled in Appendix C. As the examples provided in table 27 indicate, however, most HIV/AIDS plans do not give equal treatment to the components, and much more specificity is needed. Tables 28–30 show the level of specificity required to involve all levels of management in the application of the law as well as in the building of a more supportive work environment.

Education and Training

My study shows that CAO knowledge and attitudes about HIV/AIDS and the law can influence the level of preparedness. If so, workplace-oriented education and training can help increase preparedness. As is evident from a comparison of HIV/AIDS plans illustrated in table 27 and in Appendix C, however, the majority of municipalities fail to address the education and training needs of the workforce adequately. Although basic HIV/AIDS information is available, too often it is provided through courses or presentations at which attendance is not mandatory or simply through the distribution of posters and brochures in the employee lounge or lunchroom.[11] Furthermore, the process of training typically involves management less than it does HIV/AIDS educators brought in from outside. In addition, education often stops at superficial information without examining behavioral dimensions or the application of the epidemiology and laws to concrete workplace situations.

Few municipalities train supervisors specifically in the management of HIV/AIDS-related situations. Consequently, managers lack opportunities to gain better perspectives on reasonable accommodation issues or to learn new ways of controlling the workplace environment in the age of AIDS.

While several workplace training programs focus on the epidemiological and legal sides of the crisis, they too tend to lack specificity in applying basic principles to concrete workplace situations.[12] Training, the final component of the HIV/AIDS workplace plan, as shown in table 31, tries to correct for these problems. It requires the direct involvement of management and permits a systems approach to link it with other parts of the plan.[13] In essence, management is responsible for creating the workplace plan. Annual training sessions provide information that enables management to improve it.

Confidential, Mandatory Testing and Counseling

To be more proactive, CAOs need precise and current information about the epidemic's impact on their own workforces. Such information permits them to plan their proactivity—to gauge what must be done, to what extent, and how and when to accomplish it. City managers and mayors can use this information to calculate more accurately the costs of the retrovirus and its impact on local government's capacity to deliver services at optimal levels. In addition, access to such information

Table 27. Insufficiently Specific Municipal HIV/AIDS Plans: Selected Examples

*Component 1:   A statement supporting the civil rights of all current and prospective
                 employees who are in the HIV spectrum*

Honolulu, Hawaii

The City recognizes that some of its employees may have or may contract an
infectious/contagious disease, and that some of its prospective employees may have
such diseases. It is the City's policy that employees and prospective employees shall
not be discriminated against in employment because they have such diseases, provided
they are able to perform their jobs in a satisfactory manner without undue hazard to
themselves or others.

Sanford, Florida

Any person with AIDS, ARC, or HIV shall have every protection made available to
handicapped persons.

Component 2:   A set of procedures for dealing with HIV workers

Los Angeles, California

[Management's actions] must reflect sensitivity to the specially confidential nature of
HIV-related information. The law has very strict requirements regarding the
circumstances under which disclosure of such information may occur because of
AIDS's powerful potential for social stigma.

St. Joseph, Missouri

Supervisors need to be encouraged to confront workplace rumors. Disciplinary action
will be taken against anyone who attempts to spread rumors about, or isolate or ha-
rass, the employee with AIDS.

Component 3:   A set of services available to HIV employees

Portsmith, Virginia

Supervisors of employees who are diagnosed with lifethreatening diseases shall make
reasonable accommodations to allow employees to continue working: this may
include, among other things, changes in the physical work environment, adjustment of
job duties, or transfer to a more suitable position. Personnel and Health Department
staff are available to assist supervisors. Benefits consultation including, but not limited
to, health insurance, retirement, leave, and compensation will be provided.

Mt. Pleasant, Michigan

Job modification or transfers may be enacted: to ensure that the AIDS-infected
employee is medically fit and able to perform work and work-related tasks; or to avoid
exposure of other workers from secondary illnesses which may be contagious.

Table 27. *continued*

Component 4:   *A plan to provide education for all employees and on-going training for supervisors on managing AIDS-related situations*

North Las Vegas, Nevada

The City will sponsor and participate in ongoing AIDS education and awareness seminars. Informational materials may be obtained from the Clark County Health Department.

Kinston, North Carolina

The City of Kinston shall provide mandatory training and appropriate educational materials concerning AIDS, AIDS-related conditions and a copy of this policy in an orderly and timely manner.

---

might make management more supportive and less ambivalent toward employees in the HIV spectrum. After all, prejudices about HIV/AIDS remain unchallenged until we put specific names and familiar faces on the statistics.

For many reasons, then, HIV/AIDS-related planning and decision making cannot be based on rough guesses that underestimate the number of seropositive individuals who are employed by local government or by any other work organization. Knowing who is in the HIV spectrum seems so critical to effective management of the HIV/AIDS crisis that the acquisition of this information cannot be left to voluntary or unsystematic means. Rather, information can best be secured through routine, confidential, and mandatory HIV antibody blood testing.

As discussed in Chapter 3, the ADA and the Rehab Act prohibit mandatory testing as a screening device unless it is (1) narrowly focused, (2) job related, (3) consistent with business necessity, and (4) administered to all employees within a specific classification. The courts, national policymakers, and many scholars and AIDS advocates support this position for the very best reasons.[14] Employers might otherwise use tests to discriminate against seropositive applicants and employees who are qualified to do the job. Even a casual overview of today's news confirms that in our imperfect society prejudice finds its way into many hiring and promotion practices. Testing and reporting, however, are the only ways to place an employer on notice that specific workplace procedures and activities are legally necessary and expected. The testing of all employees would encourage seropositive individuals to exercise their rights as members of a protected group and, in so doing, to reduce the stigma associated with the retrovirus. While concern about the misuse of test results is quite valid, there is a much greater imperative to apply this kind of information to the task of improving the level of workplace preparedness in managing the HIV/AIDS crisis.

Table 28. Requisite Specificity in HIV/AIDS Plans: Civil Rights

Component 1:   *A statement supporting the civil rights of all current and prospective employees who are in the HIV spectrum*

The city of _____ understands that some of its employees and job applicants may be infected with the Human Immunodeficiency Virus (HIV) or may have Acquired Immunodeficiency Syndrome (AIDS). It is our policy to comply with all civil rights legislation, including the Americans with Disabilities Act (ADA) and the Rehabilitation Act. Employees and job applicants with AIDS or HIV shall have every protection and assistance that are available to other disabled employees and job applicants. Job applicants and employees with HIV/AIDS will not be discriminated against as long as they are otherwise qualified—possess the ability to perform the essential job functions with or without reasonable accommodations—for the positions they seek or hold. In compliance with the Rehabilitation Act, we also will take affirmative action in our hiring and promotion practices on behalf of people with HIV/AIDS.

The city of _____ also recognizes and acknowledges that:

Job applicants and employees with HIV/AIDS do not act the same, do not respond to having HIV/AIDS in the same manner, do not have identical concerns or fears, and do not need identical assistance from the organization.

Job applicants and employees with HIV/AIDS experience incredible levels of stress. They are afraid of what will happen to them and their loved ones. This is equally true for the job applicant or employee that is asymptomatic as one that has full-blown AIDS.

Job applicants and employees with HIV/AIDS may not have a strong support system outside of the workplace.

Upon receiving the diagnosis of having HIV/AIDS, the job applicant or employee may require a 3–12-month adjustment period to come to terms with the diagnosis.

Upon receiving the diagnosis of having HIV/AIDS, job applicants and employees tend to go through the five stages of death: denial, anger, bargaining, depression, and acceptance. The first three stages are most pronounced during the remaining time spent at the workplace.

People with HIV/AIDS need a sense of purpose, which is often fulfilled at the workplace.

Good employees are good employees, regardless of their HIV/AIDS status. We intend to do everything possible to keep our good employees who have contracted HIV/AIDS.

Table 29. Requisite Specificity in HIV/AIDS Plans: Procedures

Component 2:   A set of procedures for dealing with employees in the HIV spectrum

The city of _____ has established a set of procedures for assisting job applicants and employees with HIV or AIDS.

In order to receive protection and reasonable accommodations under the Americans with Disabilities Act, as well as affirmative action consideration under the Rehabilitation Act, the job applicant or employee with HIV/AIDS must provide (1) notification of the HIV/AIDS status and (2) documentation about the HIV/AIDS status. Notification can be provided verbally, but it is in the best interest of the job applicant and employee for notification to be provided in writing.

At the discretion of the job applicant or employee with HIV/AIDS, notification and documentation can be rendered to a variety of people within the (name of workplace organization) _____ including:

- the immediate supervisor
- director of human resources
  _____ (name and phone number)
- director of the employee assistance program (EAP)
  _____ (name and phone number)
- director of health services
  _____ (name and phone number)
- ADA specialist
  _____ (name and phone number)

At the discretion of the job applicant or employee with HIV/AIDS, documentation of HIV/AIDS status may be provided either by a physician appointed by the city of _____ or by a physician selected by the job applicant or employee with HIV/AIDS.

If an employee becomes exposed to HIV, the city of _____ will give the employee the option of going to a personal physician, the County Public Health Department, Planned Parenthood, or the State University for the purposes of (1) a baseline HIV antibody blood test and (2) a second HIV antibody blood test three months later. The results of both tests will be included in the employee's confidential personnel file.

Supervisors and managers are aware of many of the common physical and mental conditions that an employee or job applicant with HIV/AIDS often experiences and have been trained to assist in finding remedy and accommodation for the workplace ramifications of these physical and mental conditions. Supervisors and managers are aware that the physical and mental conditions, as well as the general HIV status, of a job applicant or employee with HIV/AIDS constitute personal issues and confiden-

Table 29. *continued*

tial matters. Supervisors and managers will respond with corresponding sensitivity in handling the HIV-related information of the job applicant or employee.

Since the city of _____ is committed to a work environment free of discrimination and harassment, supervisors and managers will take whatever steps are necessary to prevent verbal slurs, behavioral innuendos, and rumors about employees and job applicants based upon the ACTUAL OR PERCEIVED presence of HIV, or the ACTUAL OR PERCEIVED diagnosis of HIV/AIDS, in their employees. Disciplinary actions may include termination for the practice of such verbal slurs, behavior innuendos, or rumors.

Confidentiality is also guaranteed in cases where the _____ (name of workplace organization) contracts out for services rendered by counselors, physicians, etc. In cases where such confidentiality is broken, the _____ (name of workplace organization) will terminate all relevant contracts and will refrain from conducting business with the external agency or individual in the future.

Supervisors and managers are responsible for the dissemination of, and compliance with, the nondiscrimination and nonharassment policy. Violations of the policy, on the part of managers or other employees, will be grounds for disciplinary actions up to and including termination.

Refusal to work with an employee or to provide services to anyone who has been diagnosed as having HIV or AIDS shall be cause for immediate disciplinary actions up to and including termination.

Federal legislation prohibits universal mandatory screening, but it does not preclude the use of universal and confidential mandatory physical examinations as a mechanism to promote good health within the workforce. The fear of abuse may be reduced tremendously by prohibiting the use of HIV antibody blood tests during the hiring and promotion processes. That is, using test results as a condition for employment or advancement should remain illegal, and subject to litigation, unless the job-related standard can be justified. HIV antibody blood testing and counseling, however, should be included with a battery of tests administered during mandatory annual physical examinations for every employee. Information derived from the physical examinations could then be used in a preventive or prescriptive fashion for members of the workforce as well as for the purpose of workplace and organizational planning. It would promote good health and early detection of disease in all employees.

Given the high rate of false positive test results in generalized populations, employers must commit to confirming the Elisa results by using the more expensive

Table 30. Requisite Specificity in HIV/AIDS Plans: Services

Component 3:   A set of services available to employees in the HIV spectrum

The city of _____ provides a set of services to employees with HIV/AIDS. We recognize that the workplace needs of each seropositive employee will differ according to a variety of factors, including the specific job setting, the specific stage of the disease, and the particular individual. Therefore we will make every attempt to individualize services so that each HIV-infected employee may continue to be a productive worker for as long as possible.

Services and assistance include but are not limited to:

- reconstructing job descriptions for all employees so to differentiate between *essential functions* of the job and *marginal functions* of the job. This permits the city of _____ to render reasonable accommodations if needed.
- distributing copies of this HIV/AIDS plan to all job applicants and employees in the organization.
- providing facts and information about HIV/AIDS to all employees in the organization.
- providing benefit consultation on such issues as health and disability insurance, retirement, leave, and compensation.
- providing referrals to community-based agencies that provide blood testing for HIV antibodies. Employees who fear being infected with HIV/AIDS, or those who seek a second test, shall be encouraged to call during working hours the following agencies:

Co. AIDS Division	(phone number)
Planned Parenthood	(phone number)
State University	(phone number)

- providing referrals to appropriate community agencies and organizations that offer services for people with HIV/AIDS. Employees with HIV/AIDS shall be encouraged to call during working hours the following organizations:

Nearest Metropolitan HIV/AIDS Hotline	(phone number)
Local HIV/AIDS Hotline	(phone number)
Local HIV/AIDS Foundation	(phone number)
Other Local HIV/AIDS support groups	(phone number)

When requested by the job applicant or employee with HIV/AIDS, individualized and reasonable accommodations will be provided that will assist the person who is otherwise qualified to perform the essential functions of his/her job. The Americans

Table 30. *continued*

with Disabilities Act (ADA) and the Rehabilitation Act (Rehab) recognize asymptomatic employees (who are HIV+ but have no symptoms) as being *as qualified* for reasonable accommodation as employees with full-blown AIDS. Depending on the needs of each individual, as well as on the nature of the work site and the affordability of the request, reasonable accommodation may include a wide variety of actions.

Here are just a few suggestions and examples that may help the job applicant or employee with HIV/AIDS, and his/her supervisor, to come up with specific reasonable accommodations that permit the performance of essential job functions.

- Stress Reduction Measures

  Understanding of essential job functions. A review of the job description to iden-tify tasks considered *essential* and tasks considered marginal.

  Benefit consultation. A review of benefits available. Insurance plans and options, disability insurance, health care, and pharmaceutical options. A review of Sec. 4850 of the California Labor Code, which guarantees one year's full wages if the employee was infected (through blood contact) on the job and becomes unable to work. A review of the Family Medical Leave Act.

  Outside support services. Linking the individual with existing community-based support services.

  Time-outs. Brief (3–5 minutes) private *time-out* breaks occasionally during the day to help the individual to gain composure. Time-outs might use a vacant conference room, supervisor's office, or rest room stall.

  Brief break. An occasional *brief break* for a short walk outside to regain compo-sure or an opportunity to call a support group "hot line."

  Time off. Hour or half-day *time off* for appointments with physicians or therapists.

  Flextime. Flexible working hours to permit the individual to make up time for missing work due to HIV/AIDS.

  Reduced work hours. Reduction in working hours to permit the individual eventually to work part-time.

- Changes in the Physical Work Environment

  Reassignment to light duty or staff work, especially for employees in fire or public safety divisions.

  Transfer to a more suitable position. From work that is outside or involves contact with garbage or waste material.

  Work at home. Permission for the employee to conduct parts of the essential functions at home.

  Relocation of work station. Permission for employee to move work station for a variety of reasons: to avoid direct sunlight, to be nearer to the rest room, to be in a quieter area of office.

Table 30. *continued*

- Adjustment of Job Duties to Focus Solely on Essential Functions
  Reassignment of marginal functions. Transfer marginal functions to another employee.
  Assign assistant. In selected cases, the assignment of an assistant to perform the marginal functions for the employee.

- Equipment and Arrangements
  Computer equipment. Purchase of computer equipment (modems, printers, personal computers) so that the employee may perform essential work functions at home.
  Additional protective garments. Provision of additional protective garments, such as surgical masks for employees who work outside and double heavy weight gloves for employees who work in areas like waste disposal units.
  Parking arrangements. Parking arrangements that help keep the employee as healthy as possible.

- Other Ideas
  Pooling unused sick days. The pooling of all employees' unused sick days so that they can be used by employees who need them to address health needs.
  Permitting HIV/AIDS employees to snack frequently. Allowing employees with HIV/AIDS to snack at the work setting as long as frequent snacks do not interfere with the performance of the essential functions of the job. (Many people with HIV/AIDS believe that frequent and healthy snacks throughout the day can help reduce stress and maintain body weight.)
  Having healthy foods in the workplace cafeteria and food machines to enable employees with HIV/AIDS to maintain healthy eating habits at the workplace.

Western blot test. They must also commit to providing professional pretest and posttest counseling for each employee. Information about the health of individuals must also remain confidential and be disseminated on a strict "need to know" basis. Annual aggregate test results, however, should be disseminated among all workers as well as to the public at large. In this way, practitioners and citizens alike may gain a deeper appreciation of the retrovirus's impact on municipal employees and the community.

RECOMMENDATION 2: GREATER INVOLVEMENT OF THE FEDERAL GOVERNMENT

While all HIV/AIDS situations are unique and require localized responses, the burden of finding every solution simply cannot be relegated to each locality. Lo-

Table 31. Requisite Specificity in HIV/AIDS Plans: Training

Component 4:   A plan to provide education for all employees and ongoing training for supervisors in managing AIDS-related situations

The city of _____ shall provide mandatory training and appropriate educational material concerning AIDS and workplace-related issues for all employees. New employees will receive this training at the beginning of employment. This training will include (1) a review of HIV/AIDS and how it is transmitted, (2) policies pertinent to working with employees with HIV/AIDS, (3) a review and explanation of this HIV/AIDS plan.

Managers and supervisors will receive updated training on a yearly basis. Training will include the following modules:

Module 1: Understanding HIV and AIDS

The general purpose of module 1 is to familiarize managers and supervisors with (1) some of the fears and myths about AIDS that may impact workplace performance and (2) the experience of HIV-infected employees, which also impacts workplace performance.

Specific topics include:

   1. What is HIV and AIDS?
   2. Modes of transmission
   3. Progression from HIV to AIDS
   4. AIDS-related illnesses
   5. Keeping workers healthy and productive

Module 2: Managing the Workplace

The general purpose of module 2 is to familiarize managers and supervisors with ways of maintaining a productive and healthy workplace. Topics center on the Americans with Disabilities Act (ADA) and the Rehabilitation Act as applied to HIV/AIDS.

Specific topics include:

   1. ADA and the specific work setting
   2. Nondiscrimination of seropositive employees
   3. Reasonable accommodation issues and application to specific workplace and job descriptions
   4. Undue hardship issues and application to specific workplace and job descriptions.

Module 3: Building a Positive Workplace Environment

This module focuses on "supervisor-subordinate" relations and developing a positive workplace environment. Using case law in the areas of labor relations, workforce

Table 31. *continued*

management, and AIDS, as well as experiences of local HIV-challenged employees, this module familiarizes managers and supervisors with one-on-one situations.

Specific topics include:

1. ADA's requirements of self-disclosure
2. Sensitivity in dealing with seropositive employees and job applicants
3. ADA's modification of confidentiality
4. Knowledge about community-based assistance programs
5. Controlling rumors, fears, and behavior of employees who are not HIV-challenged

Module 4A: Updating the HIV/AIDS Plan

Workshop participants are divided into two groups. Supervisors participate in module 4A. Here management is given an opportunity to reassess the quality and performance of the plan. Supervisors are given an opportunity to incorporate their experience over the past year into the plan.

Module 4B: Training the Trainer about HIV/AIDS and the Workplace

Training staff participate in module 4B, which focuses on strategies for educating the entire workforce on the issue of HIV/AIDS. This module includes discussions on how to present HIV/AIDS in nonthreatening and nonoffensive ways yet in ways that are direct and provide detailed information. It also focuses on teaching the training staff to tap local expertise and resources, as well as to disseminate information in an effective manner.

Source: Adapted from Jack DeSario, Sue Faerman, and James D. Slack, *Local Government Information and Training Needs in the 21st Century* (Westport, CT: Quorum Books, 1994): 110-112; James D. Slack, "The Americans with Disabilities Act and the Workplace: Management's Responsibilities in AIDS-related Situations," *Public Administration Review* 55 (July/August 1995): 370.

cal governments need federal resources to help them. Because HIV/AIDS is a national disaster, the federal government must take the lead in facilitating proactive initiatives in individual workplaces—initiatives that will ultimately produce positive and supportive environments.

William J. Petak notes that, with all emergency management strategies, "understanding politics and the intergovernmental complexities may be of greater importance to the success of mitigation and preparedness activities than scientific knowledge."[15] Understanding the political and intergovernmental environment may be even more critical in the case of HIV/AIDS because of the social and cultural stigma so often attached to the retrovirus. Some local government practitioners, whose jobs depend in varying degrees on local political conditions, may not be able to manage this crisis effectively. Other city managers and mayors, especially those who believe their communities are insulated from the epidemic, may not want to be involved with this crisis at all. A strong federal hand may provide the needed support for the former and the necessary oversight of the latter. As with other endeavors, both carrots and sticks are called for.

Three types of federal government activities are needed to nurture higher levels of preparedness in local government and elsewhere: regulatory, distributive, and coordinative. While the focus here is on municipal governments, the severity of the HIV/AIDS crisis indicates that the following principles should apply to all work organizations in the public and private sectors.

In the area of regulatory policies, the federal government must take action on two issues by tapping the intergovernmental funding processes and the Interstate Commerce Clause to amend the Rehab Act and the ADA, respectively. First, the Rehab Act and the ADA must reflect the need for an HIV/AIDS plan in each work setting. As noted throughout this book, an HIV/AIDS plan must be adopted to ensure a supportive workplace environment and a level of preparedness. It should set forth legal expectations as well as acceptable behavior on the part of supervisors, seropositive workers, and employees not in the HIV spectrum. The federal government should require all organizations with fifteen or more full-time employees to implement either an HIV/AIDS plan or a broader disabilities plan that contains protections and services for seropositive job applicants and employees alike.

Second, federal legislation must mandate annual physical examinations, which include HIV antibody blood testing, for every municipal employee. The legislation should not be viewed as a weapon for those who wish to screen out individuals in the HIV spectrum. Rather, both the Rehab Act and the ADA should incorporate stringent and swift criminal and civil penalties for first-time abusers of the information obtained from annual physical examinations. Test results must remain confidential, and necessary justification must be provided if the results are to be used in the screening process. But the legislation should be amended to require public and private sector employers to generate proactively the kind of information that they need to anticipate and deal effectively and compassionately with the many workplace ramifications of the HIV/AIDS epidemic.

Federal government involvement is also needed in the area of distributive policies. Managing the HIV/AIDS crisis in the workplace is going to be an expensive proposition. Costs in the private sector are often easily transferred to the consumer but, given its rather fixed and limited resources, increased operating expenses are more difficult to pass on in the public sector. Additional revenues are needed to address the disaster effectively, and they should be provided through the allocation of federal taxes. The minimization of locally borne costs will make the federal government's regulatory responsibilities more palatable to practitioner and citizen alike.

Finally, the federal government must truly empower its centralized agency, the National AIDS Policy Office of the White House, giving it the responsibility of managing and coordinating all activities in the fight against HIV/AIDS. Since its creation, the office seems to have lacked clout and the ability to lead. In too many ways and in too many instances, the office has met with opposition from individuals with other bureaucratic and political interests. From the perspective of the workplace, the national AIDS coordinator must have direct and complete responsibility for assisting both employer and seropositive employee in finding and applying information and technology to concrete situations in a timely fashion. The AIDS czar should be responsible for all regulatory and distributive actions taken by the federal government. A coordinated and centralized approach is crucial if the many dimensions and ramifications of this retrovirus are to be addressed.

CONCLUSIONS

Taking local government as the case in point, this book offers a preliminary look at the complex problem of organizational preparedness in managing the workplace ramifications of HIV/AIDS. Much more research is required. As one writer has noted, "The primary focus of research in the emergency management area has been in the general area of human response and the application of technological fixes. Little has been accomplished in the development of a better understanding of public problems and finding solutions from a public policy/public management perspective."[16] This observation is especially true in the case of HIV/AIDS. While we expect research to advance our knowledge base in the medical and epidemiological areas, we must also expand our understanding of the workplace and organizational ramifications of HIV. Future public administration research should begin where this study concludes. New models are needed with greater explanatory power, as are additional cross-sectional studies and in-depth case studies. By considering issues from the point of view of seropositive employees, too, we will greatly improve our understanding of public management models. When more local governments become better prepared, we must assess implementation effectiveness and the impact of preparedness on the lives of both citizens and seropositive employees.

We can only pray that a cure for the retrovirus is soon discovered, so that studies of this nature are relegated to dusty library shelves. While the search for successful treatment continues, however, we must hope that every local government, as well as every other employer in the private and public sectors, will strive to develop and implement the necessary workplace plans and practices. Only by doing so can we ensure a more meaningful work life for individuals in the HIV spectrum and wiser use of scarce human and material resources.

While we hope and pray for a more equitable world, we must also remain cognizant of reality. The epidemic continues to spread, and the level of preparedness remains alarmingly low in most city halls. The reality of HIV/AIDS is that it represents a new kind of crisis, and the effort to resolve it must transcend ideological and political differences. Answers will not be found in traditional Democratic or

Republican standards. Effective remedies will be cast from neither liberal nor conservative molds. The spread of HIV/AIDS has only been exacerbated by the search for politically correct answers.

We need a fresh paradigm, a new way of viewing the world in the twenty-first century. The retrovirus could have one positive effect if it forced the world to rethink its approach to crisis management and to call for solutions that are more proactive and less ideological. For students of the art and science of public policy and organizational management, the construction of such a new paradigm is the ultimate challenge in the fight against the behavioral ramifications of HIV/AIDS. Indeed, the challenge awaits all of us who wish to live in a world filled with reason and compassion.

Appendix A

Questionnaire Items, 1994 Survey and 1989 Survey

1994 SURVEY INSTRUMENT

Attitudinal Items

1. I am sufficiently knowledgeable about HIV/AIDS to handle HIV/AIDS-related situations in the workplace.
2. A city employee's health condition is personal and confidential.
3. It's OK for city employees with HIV/AIDS to have direct contact with citizens.
4. Employees with "full-blown" AIDS should be terminated from the work force, regardless of their ability to do their job.
5. The city should not hire people with HIV/AIDS, regardless of their ability to perform the essential functions or tasks of the job.
6. City employees who have HIV/AIDS, but have no physical symptoms or conditions, should be given special assistance or accommodations in the workplace.
7. Citizens should not have a right to know which city department(s) have employees with HIV/AIDS.
8. As long as city employees with HIV/AIDS are able to perform the essential functions or tasks of a job, they should be treated the same as other city employees.
9. City employees suspected of being homosexual should be required to take an HIV antibody (AIDS) blood test.
10. Most citizens in my community would oppose the hiring of people with HIV/AIDS to the city's work force.
11. A city employee's personal physician should not be the source for determining the employee's capability to work.
12. The city should take precautions to protect medical information that it collects regarding a city employee's health condition.
13. HIV antibody (AIDS) blood testing should be mandatory for all new city employees.
14. City employees should have the right to have HIV antibody (AIDS) blood test results remain confidential.
15. City employees with HIV/AIDS should be given special assistance or accommodations so that they can perform their job's essential functions or basic tasks.

16. Laws should protect homosexuals from workplace discrimination.
17. Citizens should not have a right to know the identity of people with HIV/AIDS who are employees of the city.
18. City employees with HIV/AIDS should not receive special assistance or accommodations at the workplace when illnesses are in remission.
19. It should be OK to discriminate against city employees who have HIV/AIDS.
20. People with HIV/AIDS should not be protected by the Americans with Disabilities Act.
21. City employees with HIV/AIDS should not be given the same workplace assistance or accommodations as given to other disabled city employees.
22. Providing special assistance or accommodations to disabled workers will lead to the city having to cut budgets in other areas.
23. City employees with HIV/AIDS should not be separated from other employees.
24. City employees with HIV/AIDS should not have direct contact with children.
25. HIV antibody (AIDS) blood testing should not be mandatory for any city worker.
26. City policies are not adequate for handling HIV/AIDS-related situations at work.
27. HIV antibody (AIDS) blood testing should be mandatory for city employees who have direct contact with the public.
28. In my city government, there is no need to develop specific plans and procedures for dealing with HIV/AIDS in the workplace.
29. You cannot catch HIV/AIDS from casual contact with people who have HIV/AIDS.
30. Citizens do not have a right to know the number of employees with HIV/AIDS in the city's work force.
31. A city employee with HIV/AIDS has a right to continue to work as long as his/her health condition allows.
32. Laws should not allow the city to collect information regarding a city employee's health condition.
33. I am sufficiently knowledgeable about the Americans with Disabilities Act (ADA) to handle disability-related situations in the workplace.
34. City employees with HIV/AIDS should be discharged from the city work force.
35. In most cases, it will be too expensive to provide special workplace assistance or accommodations to city employees who have HIV/AIDS.
36. HIV/AIDS should not be given the same status as other long-term disabilities.

Workplace Items

1. For otherwise qualified *job applicants* with HIV/AIDS, the city is prepared to make workplace accommodations similar to those made for people with other disabilities.

2. For otherwise qualified *job applicants* with HIV/AIDS, the city is prepared to acquire or modify equipment to meet their workplace needs.

3. For otherwise qualified *job applicants* with HIV/AIDS, the city is prepared to restructure jobs to meet their workplace needs.

4. For otherwise qualified *job applicants* with HIV/AIDS, the city is prepared to provide qualified readers or interpreters to meet their workplace needs.

5. For otherwise qualified *job applicants* with HIV/AIDS, the city is prepared to modify training materials to meet their workplace needs.

6. For otherwise qualified *job applicants* with HIV/AIDS, the city is prepared to pay for all necessary workplace assistance or accommodations.

7. For otherwise qualified *job applicants* with HIV/AIDS, the city is prepared to modify the work schedules to meet their workplace needs.

8. For otherwise qualified *job applicants* with HIV/AIDS, the city is prepared to modify tests to meet their workplace needs.

9. For otherwise qualified *employees* with HIV/AIDS, the city is prepared to acquire or modify equipment to meet their workplace needs.

10. For otherwise qualified *employees* with HIV/AIDS, the city is prepared to restructure a job to meet their workplace needs.

11. For otherwise qualified *employees* with HIV/AIDS, the city is prepared to modify the work schedules to meet their workplace needs.

12. For otherwise qualified *employees* with HIV/AIDS, the city is prepared to make workplace accommodations similar to those made for employees with other disabilities.

13. For otherwise qualified *employees* with HIV/AIDS, the city is prepared to modify workplace tests to meet their needs.

14. For otherwise qualified *employees* with HIV/AIDS, the city is prepared to provide qualified readers or interpreters to meet their workplace needs.

15. For otherwise qualified *employees* with HIV/AIDS, the city is prepared to pay for all necessary workplace assistance or accommodations.

16. For otherwise qualified *employees* with HIV/AIDS, the city is prepared to transfer them to other work areas if they request such transfers.

17. For otherwise qualified *employees* with HIV/AIDS, the city is prepared to modify training materials to meet their workplace needs.

18. City employees with HIV/AIDS are eligible for disability retirement if their medical condition warrants.

19. Homosexuals are protected from discrimination in the city's workplace.

20. The city has established a voluntary HIV antibody (AIDS) blood testing procedure.

21. The city has appointed a specialist to handle all issues pertaining to the Americans with Disabilities Act (ADA).

22. The city has adopted a set of procedures for dealing with HIV/AIDS-related situations.

23. The city is prepared to investigate complaints from employees about HIV/AIDS-related discrimination at the workplace.
24. The city is prepared to provide HIV/AIDS employees with benefit consultation(s) to assist them in managing health, leave, and other benefits.
25. The city is prepared to reassign otherwise qualified employees with HIV/AIDS to vacant positions to meet their workplace needs.
26. The city is prepared to refer employees concerned about having caught HIV/AIDS to agencies which offer supportive services.
27. City council has expressed concern about the possibility of having people with HIV/AIDS employed on the city's work force.
28. The city provides information about HIV/AIDS to its employees.
29. The city provides information to employees about the Americans with Disabilities Act.
30. The city already has had to deal with an HIV/AIDS-related situation in its work force.
31. The city provides an HIV/AIDS education program for its employees.
32. The city provides training for supervisors on how to deal with employees with HIV/AIDS.
33. Mandatory HIV antibody (AIDS) blood testing is part of the city's collective bargaining agreement. If yes, list covered bargaining units. If nonapplicable, please note.

Background Questions

1. Your Age
2. Race/Ethnicity
3. Sex
4. Education/Degree
5. In general, do you see yourself as being (check one):
   _____ very liberal   _____ liberal   _____ moderate
   _____ conservative   _____ very conservative
6. Number of city employees
7. City population
8. Estimate the number of city employees who may have HIV/AIDS
9. Is your community more (check one):
   _____ rural   _____ suburban   _____ urban

1989 SURVEY INSTRUMENT

Attitudinal Items

1. HIV (AIDS) infected city employees should not be given the same considerations as handicapped city employees.

2. I am sufficiently knowledgeable about AIDS to handle AIDS-related situations in the workplace.
3. My city's policies/procedures are adequate for handling AIDS-related situations at work.
4. HIV (AIDS) infected city employees should not have direct contact with citizens.
5. HIV (AIDS) infected city employees should be separated from the rest of the work force.
6. The city should not have a right to collect information regarding a city employee's health condition.
7. The city should not hire HIV (AIDS) infected people, regardless of their ability to perform on the job.
8. As long as HIV (AIDS) infected city employees are able to meet acceptable performance standards, with no health threat to others, they should be treated the same as other city employees not infected by AIDS.
9. It is acceptable for HIV (AIDS) infected city employees to have direct contact with children.
10. Discrimination in the workplace against HIV (AIDS) infected city employees should be prohibited.
11. Citizens have a right to know which city departments have HIV (AIDS) infected people as employees.
12. Special accommodations at the workplace should be made for HIV (AIDS) infected city employees.
13. Citizens have a right to know the number of HIV (AIDS) infected employees in the city's work force.
14. City employees suspected of being homosexual should be required to take an antibody (blood) test for AIDS.
15. A city employee's personal physician should be the one to determine the employee's capability to work.
16. HIV antibody (AIDS) blood testing should not be mandatory for any city worker.
17. City workers have the right to have HIV antibody (AIDS) blood test results remain confidential.
18. In my city government, there is no need to develop specific plans and procedures for dealing with AIDS in the workplace.
19. HIV (AIDS) infected city employees have a right to continue to work as long as their health condition allows.
20. The city should take precautions to protect medical information that it collects regarding a city employee's health condition.
21. A city employee's health condition is personal and confidential.
22. HIV (AIDS) infected city employees should be discharged from the city work force.
23. HIV antibody (AIDS) blood testing should be mandatory for all new city employees.

24. AIDS should be treated as any other long-term disability.
25. HIV antibody (AIDS) blood testing should be mandatory for city employees who have direct contact with the public.
26. Citizens do not have a right to know the identity of HIV (AIDS) infected employees in the city's work force.

Workplace Items

27. The city already has had to deal with an AIDS-related situation in the city's work force.
28. The city has adopted a set of guidelines for dealing with AIDS-related situations.
29. The city provides information about AIDS to its employees.
30. The city provides an AIDS education program for its employees.
31. The city refers employees concerned about having contracted AIDS to agencies which offer supportive services for people with AIDS.
32. The city provides HIV (AIDS) infected employees with benefit consultation to assist them in managing health, leave, and other benefits.
33. HIV (AIDS) infected city workers are eligible for disability retirement if their medical condition warrants.
34. The city is prepared to transfer, to other work areas, HIV (AIDS) infected employees who request a transfer.
35. The city is prepared to transfer, to other work areas, non-HIV (AIDS) infected employees who feel threatened by a co-worker's HIV (AIDS) illness.
36. The city is prepared to develop alternative work schedules or assignments for HIV (AIDS) infected employees.
37. The city has established a voluntary HIV antibody (AIDS) blood testing procedure.
38. The city provides training for its administrators and supervisors in dealing with AIDS-related situations.
39. The city investigates complaints from employees about AIDS-related discrimination at the workplace.
40. If not covered above, please list other components of your city's AIDS policy/ procedures:

Background Items

41. Your age
42. Your race
43. Sex
44. Education/Degree
45. In general, do you see yourself as being (check one):

_____ very liberal   _____ liberal   _____ moderate
_____ conservative   _____ very conservative

46. Number of city employees
47. Current estimated number of HIV (AIDS) infected city employees
48. Estimated current population of your city
49. Would you characterize your community as being in a (check one):
    _____ rural setting   _____ urban setting

Appendix B
HIV Testing

Two types of HIV tests are approved by the U.S. Food and Drug Administration. The first type of test detects the presence of HIV antibodies in the blood and is most commonly used at AIDS clinics throughout the world. Antibodies eradicate disease-causing infectious agents and are produced by CD_4 T-cells and B-cells. Two HIV antibody tests are used in combination: the Enzyme-linked Immuno-absorbent Assay (ELISA) and the Western blot test. The ELISA is the less expensive screening test, costing approximately $25, and is the first one performed. If the ELISA produces a positive result, the Western blot test, which costs about $50, is used as a confirming test. The ELISA test is not as accurate as the Western blot and can produce a high proportion of false-positive results. That is, the ELISA by itself may indicate seropositivity when actually no HIV antibodies are present. Approximately 50 percent to 60 percent of initial positive test results are refuted by means of the confirming Western blot test.

HIV antibody testing does not detect antibodies in all blood that carries the retrovirus. Neither the ELISA nor the Western blot can identify HIV infection when the person is in the acute HIV stage. It takes typically three months for the body to produce HIV antibodies in sufficient numbers to be detectable by the ELISA and Western blot tests. These tests will also produce false-positive results when the person has a variety of medical problems or, ironically, when the person is in the final stages of the disease and lacks the CD_4 T-cells needed to trigger the production of B-cell–based antibodies.

At the three-month mark, the ELISA and the Western blot tests are about 95 percent accurate. That is, a negative test means that there is a 95 percent chance that the person is not infected with HIV. After a six-month period, test results are over 99.999 percent accurate. Any further delay in taking an HIV antibody blood test is not advisable since the results never reach 100 percent accuracy.

The second type of test, approved by the U.S. Food and Drug Administration, identifies the actual HIV p^{24} antigen rather than the development of antibodies. There are two advantages of this kind of test. First, it is not necessary to wait three months after infection before testing since the HIV p^{24} antigen is present in the body at the moment of infection. Second, test results are 100 percent accurate.

Antigen-identifying tests are not typically administered, however, for two reasons. First, the tests are comparatively expensive. At an average national cost ranging from $250 to $300 per test, they are twice as expensive as antibody procedures.

Second, most AIDS clinics lack the skills and equipment to perform the procedures. At the present time, these tests are available only at major AIDS research hospitals and organizations. Antigen-identifying tests are offered by two companies: (1) branch DNA test by the San Francisco–based Chiron Corporation and (2) polymerase chain reaction (PCR) test by the Swiss-based Roche Corporation.

Appendix C
Two Examples of Model HIV/AIDS Plans for the Workplace

EXAMPLE 1

Sources: Adapted from James D. Slack, "Managing the Workplace Ramifications of Human Immunodeficiency Virus (HIV) and Acquired Immunodeficiency Syndrome (AIDS) for Public Agencies and Health Care Facilities in the Southern San Joaquin Valley, California" (The Public Service Institute, California State University, Bakersfield, Summer 1995); and James D. Slack and Anelia Luna, "A Model Plan for Managing the Workplace Ramifications of Acquired Immunodeficiency Syndrome (AIDS) for Municipalities in Cuyahoga County and Northwestern Ohio" (Center for Governmental Research and Public Service, Bowling Green State University, November 1992).

Component 1: A statement supporting the civil rights of all current and prospective employees who are in the HIV spectrum

The city of _____ understands that some of its employees and job applicants may be infected with the human immunodeficiency virus (HIV) or may have acquired immunodeficiency syndrome (AIDS). It is our policy to comply with all civil rights legislation, including the Americans with Disabilities Act (ADA) and the Rehabilitation Act. Employees and job applicants with AIDS or HIV shall have every protection and assistance that are available to other disabled employees and job applicants. Job applicants and employees with HIV/AIDS will not be discriminated against as long as they are otherwise qualified—possess the ability to perform the essential job functions with or without reasonable accommodations—for the positions they seek or hold. In compliance with the Rehabilitation Act, we will also take affirmative action in our hiring and promotion practices on behalf of people with HIV/AIDS.

The city of _____ also recognizes and acknowledges that:

> Job applicants and employees with HIV/AIDS do not act the same, do not respond to having HIV/AIDS in the same manner, do not have identical concerns or fears, and do not need identical assistance from the organization.
>
> Job applicants and employees with HIV/AIDS experience incredible levels of stress. They are afraid of what will happen to them and their loved ones. This is as

126

true for the job applicant or employee who is asymptomatic as it is for one who has full-blown AIDS.

Job applicants and employees with HIV/AIDS may not have a strong support system outside of the workplace.

Upon receiving the diagnosis of HIV/AIDS, the job applicant or employee may require a 3–12-month adjustment period to come to terms with it.

Upon receiving the diagnosis of HIV/AIDS, job applicants and employees tend to go through the five stages of death: denial, anger, bargaining, depression, and acceptance. The first three stages are most pronounced during the remaining time spent at the workplace.

People with HIV/AIDS need a sense of purpose, which is often provided by the workplace.

Good employees are good employees, regardless of their HIV/AIDS status. We intend to do everything possible to keep our good employees who have contracted HIV/AIDS.

Component 2: A set of procedures for dealing with employees in the HIV spectrum

The city of _____ has established a set of procedures for assisting job applicants and employees with HIV or AIDS.

In order to receive protection and reasonable accommodation under the Americans with Disabilities Act, as well as affirmative action consideration under the Rehabilitation Act, the job applicant or employee with HIV/AIDS must provide (1) notification of HIV/AIDS status and (2) documentation about HIV/AIDS status. Notification can be provided verbally, but it is in the best interest of the job applicant and employee to provide notification in writing.

At the discretion of the job applicant or employee with HIV/AIDS, notification and documentation can be rendered to a variety of people within the _____ _____ (name of workplace organization), including:

- immediate supervisor
- director of human resources
  _____ (name and phone number)
- director of the employee assistance program (EAP)
  _____ (name and phone number)
- director of health services
  _____ (name and phone number)
- ADA specialist
  _____ (name and phone number)

At the discretion of the job applicant or employee with HIV/AIDS, documentation of HIV/AIDS status may be provided either by a physician appointed by the city of _____ or by a physician selected by the job applicant or employee with HIV/AIDS.

If an employee becomes exposed to HIV, the city of _____ will give the employee the option of going to a personal physician or public health agency for the purposes of (1) a baseline HIV antibody blood test and (2) a second HIV antibody blood test three months later. The results of both tests will be included in the employee's confidential personnel file.

Supervisors and managers are aware of many of the common physical and mental conditions that an employee or job applicant with HIV/AIDS often experiences and have been trained to assist in finding remedy and accommodation for the workplace ramifications of these physical and mental conditions. Supervisors and managers are aware that the physical and mental conditions, as well as the general HIV status, of a job applicant or employee with HIV/AIDS constitute personal issues and confidential matters. Supervisors and managers will respond with corresponding sensitivity in handling the HIV-related information of the job applicant or employee.

Since the city of _____ is committed to a work environment free of discrimination and harassment, supervisors and managers will take whatever steps are necessary to prevent verbal slurs, behavioral innuendos, and rumors about employees and job applicants based upon the *actual or perceived* presence of HIV, or the *actual or perceived* diagnosis of HIV/AIDS in their employees. Disciplinary actions may include termination for the practice of such verbal slurs, behavior innuendos, or rumors.

Confidentiality is also guaranteed in cases where the _____ (name of workplace organization) contracts out for services rendered by counselors, physicians, etc. In such cases, where confidentiality is broken, the _____ _____ (name of workplace organization) will terminate all relevant contracts and will refrain from conducting business with the external agency or individual in the future.

Supervisors and managers are responsible for the dissemination of, and compliance with, the nondiscrimination and nonharassment policy. Violations of the policy, on the part of managers or other employees, will be grounds for disciplinary actions up to and including termination.

Refusal to work with an employee or to provide services to anyone who has been diagnosed as having HIV or AIDS shall be cause for immediate disciplinary actions up to and including termination.

Component 3: A set of services available to employees in the HIV spectrum

The city of _____ provides a set of services to employees with HIV/AIDS. We recognize that the workplace needs of each seropositive employee will differ according to a variety of factors, including the specific job setting, the specific stage of the disease, and the particular individual. Therefore we will make every attempt to individualize services so that each HIV-infected employee may continue to be a productive worker for as long as possible.

Services and assistance include but are not limited to the following:

- reconstruct job descriptions for all employees so as to differentiate between *essential functions* of the job and *marginal functions* of the job. This permits the city of _____ to render reasonable accommodation if needed;
- distribute copies of this HIV/AIDS plan to all job applicants and employees in the organization;
- provide facts and information about HIV/AIDS to all employees in the organization;
- provide benefit consultation on such issues as health and disability insurance, retirement, leave, and compensation;
- provide referrals to community-based agencies that provide blood testing for HIV antibodies. Employees who fear being infected with HIV/AIDS, or those who seek a second test, shall be encouraged to call during working hours the following agencies:
  [list local agencies here]
- provide referrals to appropriate community agencies and organizations that offer services for people with HIV/AIDS. Employees with HIV/AIDS shall be encouraged to call during working hours the following organizations:
  [list agencies in nearest large city here]

When requested by the job applicant or employee with HIV/AIDS, individualized and reasonable accommodation will be provided that will assist the person who is otherwise qualified to perform the essential functions of his/her job. The Americans with Disabilities Act (ADA) and the Rehabilitation Act (Rehab) recognize asymptomatic employees (the status of being HIV+ without having any symptoms) as being *as qualified* for reasonable accommodation as are employees with full-blown AIDS. Depending on the needs of each individual, as well as on the nature of the work site and the affordability of the request, reasonable accommodation may include a wide variety of actions.

The following suggestions and examples may help the job applicant or employee with HIV/AIDS, and his/her supervisor, to design specific reasonable accommodations that permit the performance of essential job functions.

- Stress Reduction Measures

  Understanding of essential job functions. A review of the job description to identify tasks considered *essential* and tasks considered marginal.

  Benefit consultation. A review of benefits available. Insurance plans and options, disability insurance, health care, and pharmaceutical options. A review of Sec. 4850 of the California Labor Code, which guarantees one year's full wages if the employee was infected (through blood contact) on the job and becomes unable to work. A review of the Family Medical Leave Act.

Outside support services. Linking the individual with existing community-based support services.

Time-outs. Brief private *time-out* breaks (three to five minutes) occasionally during the day to help the individual to gain composure. Location of time-outs might be a vacant conference room, supervisor's office, or rest room stall.

Brief break. Providing an occasional *brief break* for a short walk outside to regain composure, or an opportunity to call a support group "hot line."

Time off. An hour or a half day off for appointments with physicians or therapists.

Flextime. Permitting the individual to make up time for missing work because of HIV/AIDS.

Reduced work hours. Permitting the individual to work part-time eventually.

- Changes in the Physical Work Environment

Reassignment to light duty or staff work, especially for employees in fire or public safety divisions.

Transfer to a more suitable position. From work that is outside or involves contact with garbage or waste material.

Work at home. Permitting the employee to conduct parts of the essential functions at home.

Relocation of work station. Permitting the employee to move the work station for a variety of reasons: to avoid direct sunlight, to be nearer to rest room, to be in a quieter area of office.

- Adjustment of Job Duties to Focus Solely on Essential Functions

Reassignment of marginal functions. Transfer marginal functions to another employee.

Assign assistant. In selected cases, assign an assistant to perform the marginal functions for the employee.

- Equipment and Arrangements

Computer equipment. Purchase of computer equipment (modems, printers, personal computers) for performing essential functions at home.

Additional protective garments. Individuals may want to use additional protective garments, such as surgical masks for employees who work outside or double-heavy-weight gloves for employees who work in waste disposal units.

Parking arrangements. Provide parking arrangements that help keep the employee as healthy as possible.

- Other Ideas

Pooling unused sick days. Pool all employees' unused sick days for use by employees who need them to address health needs.

Permitting HIV/AIDS employees to snack frequently. Many people with HIV/AIDS believe that frequent and healthy snacks throughout the day can help reduce stress and maintain body weight. As long as frequent snacks do not interfere with the performance of the essential functions of the job, management might consider allowing employees with HIV/AIDS to snack at the work setting.

Having healthy foods in the workplace cafeteria and food machines. Enable employees with HIV/AIDS to maintain healthy eating habits at the workplace by stocking food machines appropriately.

Component 4: A plan to provide education for all employees and ongoing training for supervisors in managing AIDS-related situations

The city of _____ shall provide mandatory training and appropriate educational material concerning AIDS and workplace-related issues for all employees. New employees will receive this training at the beginning of employment. This training will include (1) a review of HIV/AIDS and how it is transmitted, (2) policies pertinent to working with employees with HIV/AIDS, and (3) a review and explanation of this HIV/AIDS plan.

Managers and supervisors will receive updated training on a yearly basis. Training will include the following modules.

Module 1: Understanding HIV and AIDS

The general purpose of module 1 is to familiarize managers and supervisors with (1) some of the fears and myths about AIDS that may impact workplace performance and (2) the experience of HIV-infected employees, which also impacts workplace performance.

Specific topics include:

1. What is HIV and AIDS?
2. Modes of transmission
3. Progression from HIV to AIDS
4. AIDS-related illnesses
5. Keeping workers healthy and productive

Module 2: Managing the Workplace

The general purpose of module 2 is to familiarize managers and supervisors with ways of maintaining a productive and healthy workplace. Topics center on the Americans with Disabilities Act (ADA) and the Rehabilitation Act as applied to HIV/AIDS.

Specific topics include:

1. ADA and the specific work setting
2. Nondiscrimination with respect to seropositive employees
3. Reasonable accommodation issues and application to specific workplace and job descriptions
4. Issues of undue hardship and application to specific workplace and job descriptions

Module 3: Building a Positive Workplace Environment

This module focuses on "supervisor-subordinate" relations and developing a positive workplace environment. Using case law in the areas of labor relations, workforce management, and AIDS, as well as the experiences of local HIV-challenged employees, this module familiarizes managers and supervisors with one-on-one situations.

Specific topics include:

1. ADA's requirements of self-disclosure
2. Sensitivity in dealing with seropositive employees and job applicants
3. ADA's modification of confidentiality
4. Knowledge about community-based assistance programs
5. Controlling rumors, fears, and behavior of employees who are not HIV challenged

Module 4A: Updating the HIV/AIDS Plan

Workshop participants are divided into two groups. Supervisors participate in module 4A. Here management is given an opportunity to reassess the quality and performance of the plan. Supervisors are given an opportunity to incorporate their experience over the past year into the plan.

Module 4B: Training the Trainer about HIV/AIDS and the Workplace

Training staff participate in module 4B, which focuses on strategies for educating the entire workforce on the issue of HIV/AIDS. This module includes discussions on how to present HIV/AIDS in ways that are nonthreatening and nonoffensive yet direct and provide detailed information. It also focuses on teaching the training staff how to tap local expertise and resources as well as how to disseminate information in an effective manner.

EXAMPLE 2

Source: Adapted from Alan Emery, "Developing a Workplace Policy for HIV" (Washington, DC: U.S. Centers for Disease Control, March 1992), 11–13.

Policy on Life-Threatening Diseases and Disabilities

_____ does not discriminate against a qualified individual with a disability with regard to job application; hiring; advancement; discharge; compensation; training; or other terms, conditions, or privileges of employment.

Furthermore, _____ recognizes that employees with life-threatening illnesses—including but not limited to cancer, AIDS, and heart disease—and other disabilities may wish and be physically able to work a regular or modified work schedule.

_____ seeks to accommodate these employees by allowing them to work as long as they are able to perform essential job functions, with or without reasonable accommodation, provided medical evidence indicates that their conditions are not a (direct) threat to themselves or others.

While accommodating employees with life-threatening diseases and other disabilities, however, _____ also recognizes its obligations to provide a safe work environment for all employees. Therefore managers should obtain appropriate medical direction, when necessary, to ensure that an employee's condition does not pose a significant risk of substantial harm to himself/herself or to other employees.

_____ offers the following resources to assist employees and managers in dealing with these issues:

- Management and employee education and information on life-threatening illness,
- Confidential referral to supportive services for employees and dependents affected by life-threatening illnesses, and
- Benefits consultation to assist employees in effectively managing health, leave, and other benefits.

Life-Threatening Illnesses and Disabilities Guidelines for Managers

When dealing with situations involving employees with life-threatening illnesses and disabilities, managers should follow these guidelines.

Confidentiality

- Information attained as a result of a permissible medical examination must be collected and maintained on separate forms and in separate medical files and be treated as a confidential medical record.

When to Seek Assistance

- If you believe that you or other employees need information about a specific life-threatening illness, or if you need further guidance in managing a situation that involves an employee with a life-threatening illness, contact: _____ _____ .
- If you have any concern about the possible contagious nature of an employee's illness, contact _____ .
- If you are concerned that the continued presence of an employee will pose a significant risk of substantial harm in the workplace, contact _____ _____ .

Reasonable Accommodation

- Make reasonable accommodation, consistent with the business needs of the unit, for employees with life-threatening illnesses and disabilities.

  "Reasonable accommodation" refers to the company's responsibility to make modifications to help enable an otherwise qualified person, with a serious illness or other type of disability, continue to work.

  When considering a possible accommodation:

- Find out from the employee what he or she feels capable of or whether a medical or disability leave would be preferred.
- Conduct periodic evaluations to determine whether the employee remains capable of performing the essential job functions, whether the accommodation is still necessary and appropriate for the situation, whether another accommodation is needed, or whether a medical or disability leave would be more appropriate.
- Seek guidance from _____ .

Coworkers

- Be sensitive and responsive to coworkers' concerns, and emphasize employee education and information available. Give no special consideration, however, to employees who feel threatened by a coworker's illness or disability.
- Encourage employees to seek assistance from _____ for medical treatment and counseling services.

Appendix D
Selected Examples of AIDS Guidelines and Other Documentation

CATASTROPHIC ILLNESS POLICY FOR THE CITY OF MESA, ARIZONA

I. Purpose/Philosophy

The City of Mesa supports continued safe employment for all employees who are able to fully perform their job. The City strives to affirm the dignity and rights of all persons with catastrophic illnesses.

II. Policy

Employees with a known catastrophic illness who are able to meet appropriate job performance standards and whose continued employment does not pose a threat to his or her own health and safety or that of others, are assured equal employment opportunities and reasonable accommodation in their employment.

    A. Each employee of the City of Mesa is expected to treat their fellow employees with respect and dignity and to make every effort to prevent discrimination against fellow employees.

    B. Information regarding the specific medical condition of an employee is personal and shall be kept confidential, except as provided by law.

    C. Education and training programs containing accurate information about catastrophic illnesses and their transmission shall be provided to all employees. These programs shall be designed to increase employees' knowledge about catastrophic illnesses and to decrease irrational fears about exposure to catastrophic illnesses through normal, workplace contact.

    D. Insurance: Catastrophic illnesses are treated like any other life threatening condition in respect to medical coverage, long-term disability and life insurance.

III. Standards

    A. The determination as to whether a person's employment or continued employment poses a threat to the employee's own health and safety or that of others or prevents an employee from meeting job requirements is made by a physician designated by the City of Mesa and may be made in consultation with the employee's physician. The City reserves the right to require an examination by a physician designated by the City of Mesa and at the City's expense to determine if the employee's condition poses a threat to the employee's own health and safety or that of others or prevents an employee from meeting job requirements.

B. The City will take every reasonable precaution to ensure that an employee's medical condition does not present a health and/or safety threat to the employee or others.

IV. Responsibilities

A. Whenever an employee identifies herself/himself as having a catastrophic illness that affects that employee's ability to do their job, the supervisor will determine what reasonable accommodation would be needed to enable the employee to fully meet the requirements of the position.

B. The Supervisor will notify the Department Manager, who may assist in determining an appropriate course of action.

POLICY REGARDING HIV INFECTION AND CITY EMPLOYMENT AND OPERATIONS FOR THE CITY OF MINNEAPOLIS

General Policy

It is the policy of the City of Minneapolis that no employee, applicant or client shall be subjected to testing, removed from normal and customary employment status, or deprived of any rights, privileges or freedoms because of AIDS or conditions associated with Human Immunodeficiency Virus (HIV) except for clearly stated and specific medical and/or public health reasons.

For the purpose of this policy, an individual with AIDS or conditions associated with HIV infection shall be defined as follows:

- Any person diagnosed as having the medical condition known as "Acquired Immunodeficiency Syndrome" (AIDS), in accordance with the Centers for Disease Control case definition.
- Any person diagnosed as having the medical condition known as "AIDS Related Complex" (ARC) in accordance with commonly accepted clinical criteria.
- Any person who is antibody or culture positive for HIV.

Specific Policies

1. Any employee known to have AIDS or conditions associated with HIV who is able to continue safe and effective work performance shall be entitled to remain in the same job classification and work location unless the employee's physician or the City's designated employee physician makes a finding that this would threaten the health of the public, the employee, or his/her co-workers. If such a finding is made, an effort will be made to modify the employees' duties based on medical recommendations by the employee's physician and the City's employee physician. The Health Department's Medical Consultant will be consulted, as needed, to make a determination about public health reasons for any change in work status.

   Requests by an employee to not work with other employees or clients who have AIDS or conditions associated with HIV will be discouraged but will be considered on a case-by-case basis by the employee's supervisor in consultation with the City's employee physician and, if necessary, the Health Department's Medical Consultant.

2. No employee shall be required to submit to an AIDS antibody test as a condition of beginning or maintaining employment with the City of Minneapolis.

Employees who have had a significant AIDS-related work incident exposure, as defined below, shall be strongly encouraged to have an AIDS antibody test. A significant exposure occurs when infectious body fluids or tissues come in contact with a person's blood or mucous membranes. The body fluids/tissues containing the virus in infected persons are blood, semen, and deep organs. These infectious secretions must come in contact with a person's mucous membranes or directly into the person's vascular (blood) system to be defined as a significant exposure. Employees who have experienced a significant AIDS-related work incident exposure as defined here shall report the incident to their supervisor and contact the City's employee physician who will then make a decision regarding the necessity of an AIDS antibody test.

3. If an employee misses work because of an AIDS-related illness and must report to his/her supervisor or personnel officer the reason for absence, the same strict confidentiality requirements that apply to any medical disclosure shall be followed.

4. The City Health Department will plan and conduct periodic workplace AIDS presentations (in addition to those already offered all city departments) and is available upon request to present worksite presentations relating to specific employee concerns.

5. The City of Minneapolis will continue to negotiate health insurance contracts which include open enrollment with no evidence of insurability. The City will continue to provide basic life insurance coverage. No person will be required to supply information of a nature not required of all persons in City negotiated insurance packages. No modifications will be made to current disability or sick leave policies based solely on AIDS.

6. The Health Department shall review this policy at least on an annual basis and make recommendations to the City Council as needed to ensure that this policy complies with the most current epidemiologically-accepted facts about AIDS and AIDS-related conditions.

CITY EMPLOYEE AIDS POLICY FOR SEATTLE, WASHINGTON

Every City employee has the right to be free from discrimination in City employment on account of race, color, sex, sexual orientation, religion, creed, ancestry, national origin, age, marital status, political ideology, or the presence of any sensory, mental or physical handicap under the provisions of Seattle's Fair Employment Practices Ordinance (SMC 14.04). The City of Seattle recognizes that persons who have or are perceived by others to have Acquired Immune Deficiency Syndrome (AIDS) or AIDS Related Complex (ARC) or those who have tested positive for the AIDS virus antibody or who are members of one of the high risk groups are included in the protections of the Fair Employment Practices Ordinance. Department heads shall be responsible for implementing this policy.

TEN PRINCIPLES FOR THE WORKPLACE

1. People with AIDS or HIV infection are entitled to the same rights and opportunities as people with other serious or life-threatening illnesses.
2. Employment policies must, at a minimum, comply with federal, state, and local laws and regulations.
3. Employment policies should be based on the scientific and epidemiological evidence that people with AIDS or HIV infection do not pose a risk of transmission of the virus to coworkers through ordinary workplace contact.
4. The highest levels of management and union leadership should unequivocally endorse nondiscriminatory employment policies and educational programs about AIDS.
5. Employers and unions should communicate their support of these policies to workers in simple, clear, and unambiguous terms.
6. Employers should provide employees with sensitive, accurate, and up-to-date education about risk reduction in their personal lives.
7. Employers have a duty to protect the confidentiality of employee's medical record.
8. To prevent work disruption and rejection by coworkers of an employee with AIDS or HIV infection, employers and unions should undertake education for all employees before such an incident occurs and as needed thereafter.
9. Employers should not require HIV screening as part of preemployment or general workplace physical examinations.
10. In those special occupational settings where there may be a potential risk of exposure to HIV (for example, in health care), where employees may be exposed to blood or blood products, employers should provide specific ongoing education and training, as well as the necessary equipment, to reinforce appropriate infection control procedures and ensure that they are implemented.

Source: Citizens Commission on AIDS, "Responding to AIDS: Ten Principles for the Workplace," U.S. Department of Health and Human Services, Office of the Regional Manager, Office of Civil Rights, January 12, 1988.

PARTIAL JOB DESCRIPTION: ESSENTIAL AND MARGINAL FUNCTIONS, COMMUNITY SERVICES OFFICER

General Purpose

Under general supervision, enforces city ordinances and state laws regarding stray, dangerous, and nuisance domestic and wild animals; investigates complaints; patrols assigned areas; captures animals; maintains an animal shelter; performs code enforcement work as required. This code enforcement position is responsible for enforcing applicable animal control regulation in a civilian capacity with limited peace officer authority. This position will perform vehicle abatement work within established parking laws, city codes, and guidelines.

Essential Duties

Investigates complaints from the public and other agencies regarding nuisance, stray, uncontrolled, dangerous, wild, or diseased animals.

Conducts initial investigation of complaints regarding animal cruelty or neglect.

Investigates animal bites, arranging for appropriate identification and quarantine.

Explains local laws, codes, and ordinances relating to the care and control of animals, filing of complaints, and the policies of the shelter to the public.

Issues citations for violations of applicable regulations.

Patrols assigned areas of operation in city vehicles.

Captures wild, stray, and unlicensed animals and transports them for impounding.

Removes dead, injured, or dangerous animals from public and private properties.

Testifies in court regarding citations and disposition of complaints.

Assists other agencies and city departments in animal control and handling.

Maintains records and prepares daily reports.

Operates humane traps, mobile radios, and related animal control tools and equipment.

Works an assigned shift, which may vary, using own judgment in deciding course of action; is expected to handle difficult and emergency situations without assistance.

Has ability to supervise inmates in cleaning, maintenance, and operation of animal shelter.

Has knowledge of methods, equipment, and safe work practices used in the care and control of animals.

Has skill in handling, capturing, and controlling animals humanely and effectively under stressful or emergency circumstances.

Has skill in dealing tactfully and effectively with the public, including hostile and irate citizens.

Has skill in assessing animal behavior and making effective decisions regarding handling, capturing, or destroying the animal.

Has skill in identifying symptoms and behaviors associated with rabies and other common domestic animal diseases.

Has skill in reading maps and following directions.

Has skill in using sound independent judgment within established guidelines.

Peripheral Duties

Provides information to the public on care and treatment of animals.

Responds to and investigates complaints of abandoned vehicles and other code violations.

Has knowledge of basic geographical layout of the city.

Has knowledge of basic species and breeds of a variety of domestic and common wild animals.

Has knowledge of state and local laws and ordinances pertaining to the proper care and control of animals.

Has knowledge of basic record-keeping principles and practices.

Source: City of Taft, California.

Notes

Foreword

1. Linda Reynolds Broughton, "American Public Administration, Learning Theory, and AIDS" (Ph.D. diss., University of Southern California, Sacramento, 1993).

Preface

1. Ronald Bayer, "Public Health Policy and the AIDS Epidemic: An End to HIV Exceptionalism?" *New England Journal of Medicine* 324 (1991): 1500–1514.

1. The Dynamics of HIV/AIDS

1. Unfounded caution is even evident at the White House of President Bill Clinton, a self-proclaimed AIDS advocate. In 1995 White House police officers chose to wear surgical gloves in greeting a delegation of gay and lesbian elected officials.

2. T-cells are actually T-lymphocytes.

3. See Randy Shilts, *And the Band Played On* (New York: Viking Penguin, 1988), and Ronald Bayer, *Private Acts, Social Consequences: AIDS and the Politics of Public Health* (New York: Free Press, 1989).

4. As reported in "Clinton: Helms Views on AIDS 'Wrong,' " *Bakersfield Californian,* July 25, 1995, p. A-7.

5. Ronald Bayer, *Private Acts,* 140.

6. *Shuttleworth v. Broward County,* No. 85-024 (Fla. Comm. Human Relations, Dec. 11, 1985). See also *Shuttleworth v. Broward County,* No. 85-6673-CIV (U.S.D.C.S.Fla., Dec. 5, 1986).

7. For instance, see James D. Slack and Anelia Luna, "A Model Plan for Managing the Workplace Ramifications of Acquired Immunodeficiency Syndrome (AIDS) for Municipalities in Cuyahoga County and Northwestern Ohio" (Center for Governmental Research and Public Service, Bowling Green State University, Bowling Green, Ohio, November 1992); and James D. Slack, "Managing the Workplace Ramifications of Human Immunodeficiency Virus (HIV) and Acquired Immunodeficiency Syndrome (AIDS) for Public Agencies and Health Care Facilities in the Southern San Joaquin Valley, California" (Public Policy and Administration Institute, School of Business and Public Administration, California State University at Bakersfield, 1995).

8. Ronald Bayer and Gerald Oppenheimer, "AIDS and the Work Place: The Ethical Ramifications," in Christine Pierce and Donald Vandeveer, eds., *AIDS: Ethics and Public Policy* (Belmont, CA: Wadsworth, 1988), 129.

9. For further explanation, see Gerald J. Stine, *Acquired Immune Deficiency Syndrome: Biological, Medical, Social, and Legal Issues* (Englewood Cliffs, NJ: Prentice-Hall, 1995); and James D.

Slack, "AIDS Policy," in Jay M. Shafritz, ed., *International Encyclopedia of Public Policy and Administration* (New York: Henry Holt, 1997).

10. CD_4 T-cells control the cellular immune system and are needed to trigger B-cells, which control the humoral (blood and lymph) immune system.

11. Common symptoms include fever/sweats, myalgia/arthralgia (muscle pain/pain in joints), malaise/lethargy, lymphadenopathy (glandular inflammation), sore throat, anorexia, nausea, vomiting, headaches/photophobia, rashes, and diarrhea.

12. The stages of the retrovirus contribute to the role played by government (and therefore politics) in the fight against HIV/AIDS. In 1992 the federal government changed the definition of full-blown AIDS to include individuals with a CD_4 T-cell count of fewer than 200 and as a result doubled the number of people with AIDS. All federal funding to seropositive individuals, as well as to organizations serving seropositive individuals, is allocated with reference to these stages. Some funding is based on T-cell counts within the AIDS category.

13. According to Gerald J. Stine, *Acquired Immune Deficiency Syndrome,* an opportunistic disease is one "caused by normally benign microorganisms or viruses that become pathogenic when the immune system is impaired" (443). These diseases and infections do not harm most people, since the immune system is typically strong enough to prevent invasive opportunities. Some of the more common are: *Pneumocystis carinii* pneumonia, chronic cryptosporidiosis (six to twenty-six bowel movements per day, one to seventeen liters of fluids passed per day), toxoplasmosis (brain abscesses), isosporiasis, mycobacterial infection, cytomegalovirus (a virus that can affect the retina as well as kidneys, lungs, and other parts of the body), candidiasis (esophageal, bronchial, pulmonary, vaginal), oral hairy leukoplakia, recurrent salmonella bacteremia, and oral candidiasis (oral thrush). Some of the more common AIDS-related cancers are Kaposi's sarcoma, non-Hodgkin's lymphoma, and primary lymphoma of the brain.

14. Minimizing stress levels and taking care of oneself are as important to long-term survival as medical therapies and antiviral drugs. Long-term survivors of HIV/AIDS indicate that this is the positive side of the disease: they tend to change their life styles and begin to take better care of themselves. One person said that it entails doing what his mother always encouraged him to do: eat lots of fresh vegetables, say "no" to drugs, and get at least 8 hours of sleep each night. For similar reasons, it appears that many long-term survivors avoid or limit the time and energy spent in engaging in sexual activities. They also use a wide range of services, like a buddy program to provide the seropositive individual with human assistance and a meals-on-wheels program that assures the invalid seropositive individual of a hot meal three times a day.

15. While people with HIV/AIDS are living longer, the mortality rate associated with this retrovirus has brought down the average life span of Americans from 75.8 years in 1992 to 75.5 years in 1994, according to data from a study by Metropolitan Life Insurance Company, as reported in the *Bakersfield Californian,* September 1, 1995, p. A4.

16. Seropositive women are beginning to live longer than seropositive men for two reasons: (1) increasingly early detection among women and (2) women may tend to take better care of themselves. HIV-positive women who do not fit into these categories, however, such as drug-addicted prostitutes on the street, tend to live shorter lives than seropositive men.

17. Antiviral drugs refer to nucleoside analogs that block protein active in the early reproduction cycle of HIV and are generally effective until the virus develops resistance. Antiviral drugs include zidovudine or azidothymidine (AZT), didanosine (ddI), zalcitabine (ddC), stavudine (d4T), and lamivudine (3TC).

18. Protease inhibitors block a specific enzyme, protease, which is crucial to the final stages of HIV replication. Specific protease inhibitors include saquinavir, ritonavir, indinavir, and nelfinavir.

19. See Centers for Disease Control and Prevention, "AIDS Deaths Decline while Decreases Are Noted in Perinatally Acquired Cases," *HIV/AIDS Prevention* (March 1997): 5.

20. For instance, see Marisa Katz and Kim Painter, "AIDS Experts Detail Drug Standard," *USA Today,* June 20–22, 1997, p. 1A.

21. For instance, saquinavir administration requires that three capsules, spaced evenly three times in a 24-hour period, be taken on a full stomach within two hours of a high-fat (57 gram) meal. Indinavir, on the other hand, requires that two capsules, spaced evenly in a 24-hour period, be taken on an empty stomach with water one hour before or two hours after a meal.

22. The needle category includes shared instruments for the piercing of ears and the making of tattoos.

23. In the case of oral sex, for instance, the infected blood by-product in the semen must find cuts in either the mouth or the digestive system before it can enter the blood system. Similarly, infected vaginal fluids must find a cut in the skin of the penis or travel through the opening of the urethra, down the penis, into the urinary tract and through a cut into the blood.

24. Observations in this section are based on personal interviews with persons with HIV/AIDS throughout California during the spring and summer of 1995. Funding for the project was provided by the California State University at Bakersfield (University Research Council and School of Business and Public Administration).

25. For instance, a group of prostitutes in Ethiopia are believed to have contracted HIV but persistently test negative. We also cannot explain fully the reasons for long-term survival in a few seropositive individuals.

26. See Associated Press, "Clinton Sets Deadline for AIDS Vaccine," as reported in the *Bakersfield Californian,* May 19, 1997, p. A1.

27. Historians sometimes argue that burning at the stake, a technique of execution used in the Middle Ages, may have caused more pain before death than AIDS does. One would "charcoal" from the feet upward, so that the sufferer took hours, and quite frequently days, to die. This is where the phrase "put another log on the fire" originated; people would do so in order to bring about death to a friend in a more timely (hence compassionate) fashion.

Some of the symptoms of AIDS-related diseases that commonly occur simultaneously and/or sequentially include: dementia, diarrhea, abdominal pain, the enlargement of the brain, kidneys, and lungs; hallucinations; patches of hairy white tissue that can block or impair breathing; and lesions that can also block the breathing tube. In addition, bones may become brittle and joints inflamed, while feet alternate between numbness and burning. Patients may pass as many as twenty-five bowel movements per day and twenty liters of fluids per day and may experience a combination of cancers, including Kaposi's sarcoma, non-Hodgkin's lymphoma, and primary lymphoma of the brain.

28. Mark E. Wojcik, "AIDS and Funeral Homes: Common Legal Issues Facing Funeral Directors," *John Marshall Law Review* 27 (Winter 1994): 411–434.

29. Elisabeth Kübler-Ross, *Questions and Answers on Death and Dying* (New York: Collier Books, 1974); and Kübler-Ross, *On Death and Dying* (New York: Macmillan, 1969).

30. The inability to accept death occurs despite the initial feeling of immediate mortality. People who walk out of the testing center with a positive HIV test result often believe incorrectly that they will be dead within the next few days or weeks. The feeling of immediate death is so great among some who first learn of their seroconversion that physical restraint is sometimes needed before the PLWA can hear that HIV does not involve immediate death. A counselor at Planned Parenthood of Central California reported that he had to chase a client down the street who was unwilling to consider the consequences of having a positive test result.

31. The CDC estimates 1 million people, although unofficially some members of CDC fear that the number of people who do not know that they are HIV positive might be as high as 50 or 100 times the number of people who have AIDS. Members of the group AIDS Coalition to Unleash Power (ACT-UP) estimate that more than 5 million people are HIV positive. Staff at the Gay Men's Health Crisis (GMHC) suggest that the number might be over 3 million people. Some re-

searchers believe that the rate of HIV infection far exceeds 1 percent of the general population. For instance, the rate of HIV infection among sex workers has become a fair barometer of infection within the general population of a specific locality. See Constance B. Wolfsy, "AIDS and HIV Infection in Prostitutes: Epidemiology," in P. T. Cohen, Merle A. Sanda, and Paul A. Volberding, eds., *The AIDS Knowledge Base: A Textbook on HIV Disease from the University of California, San Francisco, and the San Francisco General Hospital* (Waltham, MA: Medical Publishing Group, 1990), section 1.1.19. In some metropolitan areas, such as El Paso–Juarez, 70 percent of the sex workers are seropositive. See Felipe Peralta, Patricia A. Sandau-Beckler, and Rosario H. Torres, "A Survey of AIDS Knowledge and Attitudes Among Prostitutes in an International Border Community," *Multicultural Human Services for AIDS Treatment and Prevention* 2 (1992): 71–84.

32. Because of the stigma attached to HIV/AIDS, death certificates and newspaper obituaries are not reliable sources for locating people who have died of AIDS.

2. HIV/AIDS, Public Policy, and the Public Service

1. Scott Burris, "Public Health, 'AIDS Exceptionalism,' and the Law," *John Marshall Law Review* 27 (Winter 1994): 252.

2. One exception might be multi-drug-resistant (MDR) tuberculosis.

3. In some circles of our rather macho world, evidence of venereal disease may be applauded as a sign of manhood in the teenage boy or a rite of passage for the college student in the fraternity. Although tuberculosis is a very serious and contagious disease, it is not generally associated with ostracism as is the retrovirus. Unlike any other disease we face today, HIV/AIDS jeopardizes one's lifestyle as well as one's life.

4. See Centers for Disease Control and Prevention, *HIV/AIDS Surveillance Report* 9:1 (1997): 8–10, tables 3–5. Although many seropositive Americans contracted the retrovirus through homosexual behavior, the spread of HIV/AIDS in Africa and Asia has been a result of predominantly heterosexual contact.

5. It is important to note that rights of the individual are not all weighted equally in the Bill of Rights in the U.S. Constitution. An inherent tension is readily apparent from a comparison of the rights of the individual in the First Amendment (freedom of speech and freedom to assemble) with those in the Fourth Amendment (freedom from unreasonable searches), which may place the rights of noninfected individuals in jeopardy.

6. See Randy Shilts, *And The Band Played On* (New York: Viking Penguin, 1988); and Ronald Bayer, *Private Acts, Social Consequences* (New York: Free Press, 1989).

7. See Michael L. Closen, "Introduction: HIV-AIDS in the 1990s," *John Marshall Law Review* 27: 2 (1994): 239–250.

8. Shilts, *And the Band Played On,* xxii.

9. For a review of government responses, see James D. Slack, "The Public Administration of AIDS," *Public Administration Review* 52 (January/February 1992): 77–80.

10. The delay in policy response is apparent when one compares the swift attention given to Legionnaire's disease, which affected fewer than 100 individuals.

11. It would be easy to include President Ronald Reagan in this category, but life, as well as politics, is not always so very simple and straightforward. Although Ronald Reagan was a very conservative politician, he never openly opposed homosexuality during his tenure as governor of California. In fact, several members of his staff were gay. In addition, during the Reagan administration Nancy Reagan's hairdresser was a well-known gay American. Throughout his political career, the Reagans continued to be close to gay friends from the "Hollywood days," many of whom were invited to the White House. Moreover, both Ronald and Nancy Reagan supported Elizabeth Taylor's early efforts to fight AIDS through nongovernmental efforts.

12. Shilts, *And the Band Played On,* pt. 5.

13. Shilts, *And the Band Played On,* 53–324.

14. Shilts, *And the Band Played On,* 171. Ironically, the same attitude prevails in many parts of the social sciences in the 1990s.

15. See Bayer, *Private Acts,* 20–71; and Shilts, *And the Band Played On,* pts. 2–4.

16. *Jacobson v. Massachusetts,* 197 U.S. 11 (1905), upheld the public health efforts to make smallpox vaccination compulsory in the case of epidemics. *Cleburne v. Cleburne Living Center,* 473 U.S. 432 (1985), upheld the state's obligation to address public health crises when the nature of risk to the public is great.

17. Such restrictions might be especially useful, given the potentially deadly consequences of periods of denial and anger that typically accompany knowledge of seropositivity. See Chapter 1.

18. See James D. Slack, "AIDS Policy," in Jay M. Shafritz, ed., *International Encyclopedia of Public Policy and Administration* (New York: Henry Holt, 1997). Departments that implement HIV/AIDS public policies include Health and Human Services, Housing and Urban Development, Labor, Education, Veterans Affairs, and Defense. Independent agencies that receive HIV/AIDS funding include the Health Care Financing Agency, the Social Security Administration, the Agency for International Development, and the Equal Employment Opportunity Commission.

19. Of the total federal funding budgeted for HIV/AIDS, 43 percent is allocated for medical care, 35 percent for basic research, 14 percent for education and prevention, and 8 percent for cash assistance.

20. Cultural considerations even influence epidemiological tracking. For instance, HIV-infected Catholic Mexican-American teenage girls in southern New Mexico will, for cultural reasons, quite often deny having had sexual intercourse with boyfriends. If they are pressed by public health officials, they typically admit to engaging in "backpacking," or anal sex. In the girl's eyes, backpacking enables her to maintain her virginity, a culturally important attribute, while satisfying the sexual desires of her boyfriend, a socially important task. At the same time she is using an effective form of birth control and feels able to deny that she actively engages in sexual intercourse because, from her perspective, the boy is doing all the work in the act of backpacking.

21. On civil liberties concerns, see, for instance, Kristine M. Gibbie, "The President's Commission on AIDS: What Did It Do?" *American Journal of Public Health* 79 (July 1989): 868–870. For the opposing viewpoint, see William E. Dannemeyer and Michael G. Franc, "The Failure of AIDS Prevention Education," *Public Interest* 96 (Summer 1989): 47–60.

22. For a review, see Bayer, *Private Acts,* 147–153.

23. June E. Osborn, "AIDS: Politics and Science," *New England Journal of Medicine* 318 (February 18, 1988): 446.

24. See Walter J. Jones and James A. Johnson, "AIDS and the Workplace: Legal and Policy Considerations for Personnel Managers," *Review of Public Personnel Administration* 9 (Summer 1989): 3–14.

25. Jones and Johnson, "AIDS and the Workplace," 6.

26. It is estimated that one in twelve small businesses has an employee who is within the HIV spectrum. See Susie Stephenson, "Dealing with AIDS: AIDS in the Workplace," *Restaurants and Institutions* 104:8 (April 1, 1994): 66.

27. For an excellent and concise review of fear associated with HIV/AIDS, see David Schulman, "AIDS Discrimination: Its Nature, Meaning, and Function," *Nova Law Review* 12:3 (Spring 1988): 1113–1140.

28. For instance, the New York City Department of Health claims that no one has ever contracted HIV from, or through, a paper cut on the hand.

29. Judith Wilson Ross, "Ethics and the Language of AIDS," in Christine Pierce and Donald Vandeveer, eds., *AIDS: Ethics and Public Policy* (Belmont, CA: Wadsworth, 1988), 39.

30. The commercial names for this drug are Bactrim and Septra.

31. If foscarnet is prescribed for CMV, the annual cost ranges from $1,600 to $2,600.

32. Remune is manufactured by Immune Response Corporation. Vistide is made by Gilead Sciences. As of 1997, Remune and Vistide were approved for general distribution by the U.S. Food and Drug Administration. Recent interviews with PLWAs in California suggest that the cost of pharmaceuticals has no ceiling. A wealthy individual in Los Angeles, for instance, spent more than $1 million annually on drugs during the four years between the time when his CD_4 T-cell count dropped below 400 until the time of his death. A Riverside resident with AIDS, gifted in the craft of carpentry, built a five-by-three-foot medicine cabinet into a wall in his bedroom in order to have sufficient space for the drugs he takes.

33. Experience in treating HIV/AIDS is perhaps the most important factor. Many PLWAs in Bakersfield, California, a metropolitan area of 300,000 people, choose to make the two-hour trek over the Tejon Pass into Los Angeles for treatment rather than use services provided at the only AIDS clinic in Kern County. Similarly many PLWAs in Columbus, Ohio, a city of 700,000 people, choose to travel two hours up I-71 to Cleveland in order to receive treatment at more experienced facilities, including the university hospitals of Case Western Reserve University and the world-renowned Cleveland Clinic. The end result of frequent long-distance traveling is further depletion of the immune system, but PLWAs who see inexperienced medical practitioners risk inadequate diagnosis and treatment.

34. Robert A. Hiatt, Bruce Fireman, Charles P. Quesenberry, Jr., and Joseph V. Selby, "The Impact of AIDS on the Kaiser Permanente Medical Care Program (Northern California Region)" (Health Program, Office of Technology Assessment, U.S. Congress, Washington, D.C., July 1988).

35. Estimated expenses acquired from the CDC "Information Desk."

36. It is an understated, conservative estimate because the model assumes a relatively low salary, includes a relatively low figure (20 percent) for contributions to sick days from non-health-care fringe benefits, and does not include temporary employee replacement costs for individuals using sick days. In addition, it does not include the cost of permanent replacement after the death of the individual. The impact of new protease inhibitors on life expectancy is also not taken into consideration. All of these factors may increase workplace costs.

37. Job Accommodation Network, 809 Allen Hall, P.O. Box 6122, Morgantown, WV 26507-9984. Tel. (800) 526-7234.

38. According to Irene Rubin, Northern Illinois University, and Sylvester Murray, Cleveland State University, these averages appear roughly accurate for the rest of the country.

39. For instance, one seropositive employee in a workplace of 100 total employees will affect the rate of utilization more than one seropositive employee in an organization with 1,000 workers.

40. For instance, see *Frank Greenberg, Executor v. H&H Music Company,* No. 91-1283 (La. Ct. App. Nov. 1991).

41. For instance, see *EEOC v. Tarrant Distributors,* No. H-94-3001 (D.S. Tex. Oct. 11, 1994); and *EEOC v. Connecticut Refining Co.,* EEOC Charge No. 161-93-0253 (Mar. 9, 1994). There have also been several out-of-court settlements pertaining to union health packages. See *Philadelphia Daily News,* July 5, 1995, p. 3.

42. For more information, contact the San Francisco AIDS Hotline and the New York–based Gay Men's Health Crisis.

43. For this reason many counseling groups, such as the Cleveland-based AIDS Taskforce, advise people to go to testing sites where only anonymous procedures are offered.

44. Observations made by a counselor at the San Francisco AIDS Hotline, June 27, 1997.

45. *Health Insurance Association of America v. Corcoran,* No. 56959 (N.Y. App. Div. Feb. 15, 1990).

46. Both CARE and HOPWA funds are currently being scrutinized by Congress. Further cuts in federal spending in this area are anticipated.

47. As of 1997, states included here are California, Connecticut, Delaware, Georgia, Illinois,

Maine, Maryland, Michigan, Minnesota, Missouri, New Jersey, New York, North Carolina, Ohio, Pennsylvania, Rhode Island, and Wisconsin.

48. Here the terms "public service," "bureaucracy," and "public administration" are used interchangeably to denote the administrative branch of government.

49. Woodrow Wilson, "The New Meaning of Government," *Women's Home Companion* 39 (November 1912), as reprinted in *Public Administration Review* 44 (May/June 1984): 195.

50. Wilson, "The New Meaning of Government," 195.

51. Services may also diminish because of costs incurred when government functions as the custodian of people with HIV/AIDS. This statement seems particularly true in the case of prisons. For instance, in California it is estimated that one prisoner of every ten is seropositive. For instance, see Tamara Koehler and Scott Forter, "Sick Prisoners Barred from Last Wishes," *Bakersfield Californian,* July 3, 1995, pp. A1–A2. The fact that more than seven thousand senior citizens have HIV/AIDS also places an unexpected burden on government. See Jane Gross, "Elderly Often are Forgotten in Battle to Control AIDS," as reported in the *Bakersfield Californian,* March 16, 1997, p. A13.

52. Of the 18.3 million government employees, 60 percent work in the local public sector, 23 percent work for state governments, and 17 percent are federal employees (U.S. Bureau of the Census, *Public Employment 1990,* Series 90-1, p. vi).

53. Calculations presume that municipal and county workers comprise 60 percent of the total public sector workforce of 18.3 million people.

54. In the Cleveland area, for instance, a group of suburban public works employees were hesitant to enter sewer tunnels because of fear that the research hospitals "up the line" were disposing the retrovirus improperly by dumping it down drains.

55. This concern is evident in the current procedure for handling cuts and nosebleeds at athletic events.

56. Members of ACT-UP have been known to toss vials of infected blood at symbols of authority.

57. The possibility of transmission increases if either the lifeguard or the child has used dental floss that day, has had dental work recently, has common (canker) sores on the lips or inside the mouth that may break and bleed, or has a missing or loose tooth.

58. For instance, see William J. Petak, ed., "Emergency Management: A Challenge for Public Administration," *Public Administration Review* 45 (January 1985): 1–172 (special issue).

59. The issue of testing and knowing who is seropositive is emerging rapidly in the area of county government licensing of foster parents.

60. Frederick C. Mosher, *Democracy and the Public Service* (New York: Oxford University Press, 1982), 8.

61. Frank J. Thompson, *Personnel Policy in the City* (Berkeley: University of California Press, 1975), 6.

62. James M. Kouzes and Barry Z. Posner, *The Leadership Challenge* (San Francisco: Jossey-Bass, 1990), 6.

3. HIV/AIDS and the Law

1. As of 1997, for instance, the state of California has enacted more than eighty pages of statutes dealing with HIV/AIDS. Los Angeles enacted the first HIV/AIDS discrimination ordinance in the nation in 1985. For a review of efforts in Los Angeles, see David Schulman, "AIDS, the Law and Society: Fact vs. Fear," *Los Angeles Lawyer* 11:6 (September 1988): 19–29.

2. The Rehabilitation Act of 1973, 29 U.S.C. sections 701–796 (1985); the Americans with Disabilities Act of 1990, 42 U.S.C. sections 12101–12211 (1995). The Rehabilitation Act is clarified

as it relates to seropositive issues by provisions of the 1988 Civil Rights Restoration Act; see 29 U.S.C. section 706(8) subparagraph (C), (1985).

3. Because of verification requirements, discussed below, people who are in the acute HIV stage are not protected by either act.

4. For an expanded discussion of the Rehabilitation Act and the ADA, see Gary S. Marx and Gary G. Goldberger, *Disability Law Compliance Manual* (Boston: Warren, Gorham and Lamont, 1991); Brenda T. Strama, ed., *AIDS and Governmental Liability: State and Local Government Guide to Legislation, Legal Issues, and Liability* (Chicago: American Bar Association, 1993); Michael Starr, "AIDS in the Workplace: Issues for Employers," *Public Management* 76:4 (April 1994): 8–25; and Michael D. Esposito and Jeffrey E. Myers, "Managing AIDS in the Workplace," *Employee Relations Law Journal* 9:1 (June 22, 1993): 3–27.

5. See 45 C.F.R. section 84.3 (1995).

6. This interpretation has been upheld in several court cases, including *Doe v. New York University,* 666 F.2d 761 (1981), and *Thomas v. Atascadero Unified School District,* 662 F.Supp.376 (C.D.Cal. 1987).

7. "Covered entity" may include more than simply a person's employer. A recent court ruling determined that agents that control health care benefits for employees may also be considered a covered entity. See *Carparts Distribution Center Inc. v. Automotive Wholesaler's Association of New England,* No. 93-1954, (Cal.Ct.App. Oct. 12, 1994), *rev'g* 62 L.W. 2083 (D.C.N.H. July 19, 1983).

8. See 42 U.S.C. 12111(5) (1995). There are some exceptions to coverage: the federal government, American Indian tribes, and bona fide private membership clubs that enjoy 501(c) status with the Internal Revenue Service. Neither labor organizations nor nonprofit and not-for-profit organizations are exempt. Many organizations that employ people only on a seasonal basis, for less than twenty weeks per year, are also not covered by the ADA. Also see U.S. U.S.C. 12113 section 103(c) (1995), which deals with specific situations in which religious entities are exempted.

9. For more discussion of these differences, see James D. Slack, "Disability Discrimination," in Jay M. Shafritz, ed., *International Encyclopedia of Public Policy and Administration* (New York: Henry Holt, 1997).

10. See 41 C.F.R. section 60-741.4 (1995).

11. See 42 U.S.C. 12101(b)(1) (1995).

12. See 41 C.F.R. sections 60-741.1–60-741.54 (1995).

13. See Executive Order No. 12,250, 45 Fed. Reg. 72995 (1980).

14. See 42 U.S.C. 12177 section 107 (1995).

15. See 36 C.F.R. pt. 1190 (1994).

16. See 42 U.S.C. 12181 section 301(9) (1995).

17. To determine whether or not the structural modifications would be "readily achievable," the ADA requires that the following factors be taken into consideration: "(A) the nature and cost of the action needed under this Act; (B) the overall financial resources of the facility or facilities involved in the action; the number of persons employed at such facility; the effect on expenses and resources, or the impact otherwise of such action upon the operation of the facility; (C) the overall financial resources of the covered entity; the overall size of the business of a covered entity with respect to the number of its employees; the number, type and location of its facilities; and (D) the type of operation or operations of the covered entity, including the composition, structure, and functions of the work force of such entity; the geographic separateness, administrative or fiscal relationship of the facility or facilities in question to the covered entity." See 42 U.S.C. 12181 section 301(9)(A)(B)(C)(D) (1995).

18. For example, the west Texas community of Coahoma, population 1,500, has rejected all federal funding since the mid-1970s.

19. Because the definitions are identical, I will henceforth use the term "disability."

20. See 42 U.S.C. 12102 Section 3(2)(A)(B)(C) (1995). Also see EEOC, *Interpretive Guidelines*, 56 Fed. Reg. 35,740 (July 26, 1991); Report of the Senate Comm. on Labor and Human Resources on the Americans with Disabilities Act of 1989, S. Rep. No. 116, 101st Cong., 1st Sess. 21 (1989); Report of the House Comm. on Education and Labor on the Americans with Disabilities Act of 1990, H.R. Rep. No. 485, 101st Cong., 2d Sess., pt. 2 at 27 (1990).

21. *Doe v. Charlotte Memorial Hospital,* Complaint No. 04-84-3096 (Health and Hum. Serv. Office of Civil Rights filed August 5, 1986).

22. *School Board of Nassau County, Fla. v. Arline,* 480 U.S. 273 (1987).

23. *Thomas v. Atascadero Unified School District,* 662 F.Supp. 376 (C.D. Cal. 1987).

24. *Thomas v. Atascadero Unified School District,* at 18.

25. *Chalk v. U.S. District Court, Central District of California,* 840 F.2d 701 (9th Cir. 1988).

26. *Leckelt v. Board of Commissioners of Hospital District No. 1 et al.,* 714 F.Supp. 1377 (E.D. La. 1989).

27. See Report of the House Comm. on Education and Labor on the Americans with Disabilities Act of 1990, at 22. See also 136 *Cong. Rec.* S9697 (July 13, 1990).

28. See 29 C.F.R. section 1630.2(i) (1995).

29. See 29 C.F.R. section 1630.2(j)(2) (1995). According to EEOC *Interpretive Guidelines* (see 56 Fed. Reg. 35,741 [July 26, 1991]): "The term 'duration' as used in this context, refers to the length of time an impairment persists, while the term 'impact' refers to the residual effects of an impairment. Thus, for example, a broken leg that takes eight weeks to heal is an impairment of fairly brief duration. However, if the broken leg heals improperly, the 'impact' of the impairment would be the resulting permanent limp. Likewise, the effect on cognitive functions resulting from a traumatic head injury would be the impact of that impairment."

30. Individuals in the acute HIV stage are excluded for reasons discussed in Chapter 1. There are simply insufficient levels of HIV antibodies present for a positive test at this stage. Without a finding of HIV antibodies, everyone with mononucleosis-like symptoms could claim to have a disability.

31. Protection for people in the asymptomatic stage of the retrovirus is underscored in 29 C.F.R. section 1630.2(1) (1995). Also see EEOC, *Interpretive Guidelines,* 56 Fed. Reg. 35,742 (July 26, 1991).

32. For the Rehab Act, see 41 C.F.R. section 60-741 (1995). For the ADA, see 56 Fed. Reg. 35,748 (July 26, 1991).

33. See EEOC, *Interpretive Guidelines,* 56 Fed. Reg. 35,749 (July 26, 1991). Also see *Fong v. U.S. Department of Treasury,* 705 F.Supp. 41 (DDC 1989); and *R.G.H. v. Abbott Laboratories,* No. 93 C 4361 (D.No.Ill. Feb 14, 1995).

34. The language quoted here is the same throughout most of both pieces of legislation. The similarity is not accidental: the ADA was passed to extend the Rehab Act to the private sector. For the Rehab Act, see 29 C.F.R. section 1613.702(f) (1995). For the ADA, see 42 U.S.C. 12111 section 101(8) (1995). Also see *Guinn v. Bolger,* 598 F.Supp. 196 (D.D.C. 1984).

35. For an excellent review, refer to Gary S. Marx and Gary G. Goldberger, *Disability Law Compliance Manual* (Boston: Warren, Gorham and Lamont, 1991); Scott Burris et al., *AIDS Law Today: A New Guide for the Public* (New Haven, CT: Yale University Press, 1993); Harold L. Hirsh, "Social, Legal, Medical, and Ethical Challenges of HIV Infection, Part 1," *Medical Trial Technology Quarterly* 39 (1993): 324; and Harold L. Hirsh, "Social, Legal, Medical, and Ethical Challenges of HIV Infection, Part 2," *Medical Trial Technology Quarterly* 39 (1993): 461.

36. EEOC regulations at 29 C.F.R. section 1630.2(n)(2)(i)–(iii) (1995).

37. For the Rehab Act, see 41 C.F.R. sections 60-741.4(a) (1995). For the ADA, see 56 Fed. Reg. 35,731 (July 26, 1991).

38. See 42 U.S.C. 12112 section 102(b)(6) (1995). Also see EEOC regulations at 29 C.F.R. section 1630.10 (1995).

39. Criteria for choosing screening devices are also relevant to the issues of reasonable accommodation and undue hardship, which are discussed below.

40. For other examples, see EEOC, *Interpretive Guidelines,* 56 Fed. Reg. 35,751–35,752 (July 26, 1991).

41. Ibid. Also see EEOC, *Interpretive Guidelines,* 56 Fed. Reg. 35,749 (July 26, 1991).

42. For instance, see *Department of Labor, OFCCP v. Texas Indus., Inc.* Fair Empl. Prac. Cas. (BNA) 18 (D.O.L. 1988).

43. Necessarily reasonable accommodations might also be available to assist the job applicant to perform the essential functions of the job adequately.

44. For other examples, refer to EEOC, *Interpretive Guidelines,* 56 Fed. Reg. 35,751–35,752 (July 26, 1991).

45. Observations based on personal interviews of Californians with HIV/AIDS about their experience in the workplace and seeking work. The project was funded by the California State University at Bakersfield (University Research Council and School of Business and Public Administration).

46. Adapted from Brenda T. Strama, ed., *AIDS and Governmental Liability* (Chicago: American Bar Association, 1993), app. A, which is based on material originally published in the EEOC *Technical Assistance Manual.*

47. See 42 U.S.C. 12112 section 102(c)(2) (1995).

48. The probable exceptions would be those positions that do not involve physical tasks as essential functions: office staff, dispatchers, budget specialists, etc.

49. 42 U.S.C. 12112 section 102(c)(3)(A)–(C) (1995). Exceptions to the confidentiality rule include: supervisors/managers, first aid and safety personnel, and governmental officials investigating claims of discrimination. See 42 U.S.C. 2112 section 102(c)(3)(i)–(iii).

50. EEOC, *Interpretive Guidelines,* 56 Fed. Reg. 35,751 (July 26, 1991).

51. For an excellent review, see Mary Anne Bobinski and William S. LeMaistre, "HIV Testing and Confidentiality," in Brenda T. Strama, ed., *AIDS and Governmental Liability* (Chicago: American Bar Association, 1993).

52. For instance, see Jack P. DeSario and James D. Slack, "The ADA and Refusals to Provide Medical Care to Persons with HIV/AIDS," *John Marshall Law Review* 27 (Winter 1994): 347–362; Sheila Taub, "Doctors, AIDS, and Confidentiality," *John Marshall Law Review* 27 (Winter 1994): 331–346; and William Adams, "The Dilemma for Minors Seeking HIV-Testing and Treatment," *John Marshall Law Review* 27 (Winter 1994): 493–512. There is also the chance of misdiagnosis. For instance, see *Chizmar et al. v. Scott P. Mackie, M.D.* 896 P.3d 196 (Alas. 1995).

53. See *Skinner v. Railway Labor Executives Association,* 489 U.S. 602, 616–618 (1989); and *Schmerber v. California,* 384 U.S. 757 (1966). For excellent reviews of this issue, see Mary Anne Bobinski and William S. LeMaistre, "HIV Testing and Confidentiality," in Strama, *AIDS and Governmental Liability;* Jean R. Sternlight, "Mandatory Non-Anonymous Testing of Newborns for HIV," *John Marshall Law Review* 27:2 (Winter 1994): 373–410; and William Adams, "The Dilemma for Minors Seeking HIV-Testing and Treatment," *John Marshall Law Review* 27:2 (Winter, 1994): 493–512.

54. For instance, see Center for Employment Relations and Law, College of Law, Florida State University, *Employment Relations Bulletin* 8 (March 1990): A-2.

55. The decision to test employees in the State Department and the Foreign Service was upheld in *Local 1812, American Federation of Government Employees v. United States Department of State,* 662 F.Supp. 50 (D.D.C. 1987).

56. For instance, see *Anonymous Fireman v. City of Willoughby,* 779 F. Supp. 402 (N.D. Ohio 1991).

57. In *Doe v. District of Columbia,* No. 91-1642 (D.D.C. 1992), 61 U.S.L.W. 2022 (July 1992), for instance, a federal court ruled that the District of Columbia violated the Rehab Act when it

withdrew an offer of employment from a firefighter applicant after he disclosed his HIV status. In *Severino v. North Fort Myers Fire Control District,* 935 F.2d 1179 (Cal.Ct.App. 1991), the court held that transfer to "light work" is a reasonable accommodation for a firefighter.

58. Walter J. Jones and James A. Johnson, "AIDS in the Workplace: Legal and Policy Considerations for Personnel Managers," *Review of Public Personnel Administration* 9 (Summer 1989): 5.

59. For the Rehab Act, see 41 C.F.R. section 60-741.2 (1995). For the ADA, see 42 U.S.C. 12111 section 101(9) (1995). For an excellent review, see Jeffrey O. Cooper, "Overcoming Barriers to Employment: The Meaning of Reasonable Accommodation and Undue Hardship in the Americans with Disabilities Act," *University of Pennsylvania Law Journal* 139:5 (May 1991): 1423–1468.

60. See *Educational Testing Service v. Liberty Mutual Fire Insurance Co.* No. C-96-2790-VRW (N.D.Cal. 1997).

61. For one court's ruling, see *Hall v. U.S. Postal Serv.,* 857 F.2d 897, 902–903 (7th Cir. 1978).

62. The Job Accommodation Network can be reached at West Virginia University, P.O. Box 6122, Morgantown, WV 26507-9984. Its telephone number is (800) 526-7234. Two outreach units that stand out for such expertise are: the Public Service Institute at California State University, Bakersfield, and the Center for Governmental Research and Public Service at Bowling Green State University in Bowling Green, Ohio.

63. See EEOC, *Interpretive Guidelines,* 56 Fed. Reg. 35,744, 35,748 (July 26, 1991); and House Comm. on Jud. Report at 40; Senate Comm. on Labor and Human Resources at 35; Report of the House Comm. on Education and Labor at 66; Report of the House Comm. on Education and Labor at 67.

64. Gary S. Marx and Gary G. Goldberger, *Disability Law Compliance Manual,* section 3.03.

65. See 42 U.S.C. 12111 section 101(9) (1995). Transfers for employees, but not for job applicants, are also permissible. See *Buckingham v. United States,* 93 C.D.O.S. 5303.

66. Thrush is yeast found in the mouth, esophagus, and vagina. Toxoplasmosis causes headaches, lethargy, confusion, seizures, fevers, and a mental slowing down. MAC causes fevers and chills, wasting, abdominal pain, diarrhea, and malnutrition due to malabsorption of vitamins and minerals. Tuberculosis can be found in the lungs, internal organs, bones, lymph glands, nerves, rectum, and brain and causes fevers, wasting, and weakness. CMV can cause blindness, fevers, diarrhea, abdominal pain, and ulcers in the esophagus, stomach, and intestinal tract. Shingles can cause extremely painful skin lesions, oral ulcers, rectal bleeding, pain, and discharge. For an excellent review, see Cohen, Sande, and Volberding, eds., *The AIDS Knowledge Base.*

67. Most commonly nausea, diarrhea, and myelopathy or numbness in the feet and hands.

68. *Alexander v. Choate,* 469 U.S. 287 (1985).

69. 42 U.S.C. 12111 section 101(1)(A) (1995).

70. 42 U.S.C. 12111 section 101(10)(B) (1995).

71. See EEOC, *Interpretive Guidelines,* 56 Fed. Reg. 35,744–35,745 (July 26, 1991). Also see Senate Comm. on Labor and Human Resources Rep. at 35; House Comm. on Education and Labor at 67. Also see *Estate of William Beringer, M.D. v. Medical Center of Princeton,* 249 N.J. Super. 597 (Law Div. 1991).

72. See EEOC, *Interpretive Guidelines,* 56 Fed. Reg. 35,744–35,745 (July 26, 1991). Also see Gary S. Marx and Gary G. Goldberger, *Disability Law Compliance Manual* (Boston: Warren, Gorham, and Lamont, 1991).

73. See EEOC, *Interpretive Guidelines,* 56 Fed. Reg. 35,752 (July 26, 1991); and 56 Fed. Reg. 35,733 (July 26, 1991).

74. *Chrysler v. DILHR,* 14 Fair Empl. Prac. Cases (BNA) 344 (Wis.Cir.Ct. 1976).

75. *Western Weighing Bureau v. DILHR,* 21 Fair Emp.Prac.Cases (BNA) 1733 (Wis.Cir.Ct. 1977).

76. *Sterling Transit Co. v. FEPC,* 121 Cal.App.3d 791, 175 Cal.Rptr. 548 (1981).

77. *E. E. Black, Ltd. v. Marshall,* 497 F.Supp. 1088 (D.Hawaii 1980).

78. *McDermott v. Xerox,* 65 N.Y. 2d 213, 480 N.E. 2d 695, 491 N.Y.S. 2d 106 (1985).

79. Indeed, courts have favored employees so much that some employers are now beginning to use alternative dispute resolution techniques to resolve disagreements regarding reasonable accommodation. See "ADR Used in Complying with Disabilities Act," *New Jersey Lawyer,* October 10, 1994, p. 40.

80. *Clarence B. Cain v. Joel Hyatt* (E.D.Pa. 1990).

81. Possible exceptions may include municipal programs using predominantly volunteers that are funded substantially by "soft monies" from private foundations and individual contributions.

82. See Chapter 2.

83. *Clarence B. Cain v. Joel Hyatt* (E.D.Pa. 1990).

84. For instance, see Mark S. Senak, "HIV Tests Must Stay Anonymous," *Los Angeles Times,* March 13, 1995, p. B-5.

85. The courts have long considered the right to privacy to be implicit in the Bill of Rights, specifically in the First Amendment (freedom of speech/communication), the Fourth Amendment (unreasonable searches), the Fifth Amendment (self-incrimination), the Eighth Amendment (cruel and unusual punishment), and the Fifth and Fourteenth Amendments read together (liberty and due process). For an excellent review, see Charles Dale et al., "Blood Testing for Antibodies to the AIDS Virus: The Legal Issues," in Norman Quist, ed., *AIDS Legal, Legislative, and Policy Issues* (Frederick, MD: University Publishing Group, 1989).

86. *Whalen v. Roe,* 429 U.S. 589 (1977), which dealt with physicians' reporting to the state of New York of the names of patients who had been prescribed Schedule II drugs; and *Thornburgh v. American College of Obstetricians and Gynecologists,* 476 U.S. 747 (1986), which dealt with the reporting of personal information on abortion patients. For an excellent review, see Bobinski and LeMaistre, "HIV Testing"; and *AIDS: The Constitution and Public Health* (Cleveland: Cleveland-Marshall College of Law, 1988).

87. *Saxton v. Vanzant,* No.26-CIV-59 (Fayette Cty., Ohio Ct.C.O., March 7, 1986).

88. *Little v. Bryce,* 44 EPD Case 37,330 (Tex.Ct.App.).

89. *Doe v. Borough of Barrington,* 729 F.Supp.376 (D.N.J. 1990), which dealt with the disclosure of information about a person with HIV/AIDS as a result of a police search.

90. *Caspary v. the State of Washington,* No. 36689-Z-I 85 (Wash.Ct.App. 1018, 1997).

91. This potential impact is acknowledged in the language of the ADA, in 42 U.S.C. 12112 section 102(c)(3)(B) (1995).

92. The definition of wrongful disclosure will vary even from state to state. California, for instance, prohibits employers from seeking information about HIV/AIDS in providing reasonable accommodation. In that state, an employee is obligated to report and document only functional consequences of disabilities in seeking reasonable accommodation. While the state's provisions in this area seek to protect the individual in the "traditional" perspective of confidentiality, some observers believe they fail to accomplish their purpose and reduce employers' ability to provide effective accommodations in some cases.

93. *Doe v. Septa,* 72 F.3d 1133 (U.S. App. 3d D, 1995). Employees trying to keep information about the seroconversion from the organization should know that filing claims for AZT will commonly cause notice in the insurance office. Even using the generic term retrovir will sometimes trigger suspicion.

94. For instance, see Jack P. DeSario and James D. Slack, "The ADA and Refusals to Provide Medical Care to Persons with HIV/AIDS," and D. H. J. Hermann, "Liability Related to Diagnosis and Transmission of AIDS," *Law, Medicine, and Health Care* 15 (Summer 1987): 165–183.

95. For instance, see "Job Safety, OSHA Berated by Industry Representatives at House Oversight Subcommittee Hearing," *Daily Report for Executives: BNA,* February 17, 1995, p. A-33.

96. For instance, *Jacobson v. Massachusetts,* 197 U.S. 11 (1905), upheld compulsory smallpox

vaccinations in the case of an epidemic. *Cleburne v. Cleburne Living Center,* 473 U.S. 432 (1985), upheld the state's obligation to address public health crises when the nature of risk to the public is great.

97. There is a rise of "AIDS phobia" claims in the 1990s. See Janine Fiesta, "HIV Legal Update, Part 2," *Nursing Management,* 27:1 (November 1996): 18–19; and Leo T. Crowley, "AIDS-Phobia Claims and the Disabilities Act," *New York Law Journal,* October 20, 1994, p. 4. Naturally AIDS phobia is not confined to the workplace. Marvin McClendon, a high school sophomore, was convicted of murdering two homosexuals. He claimed that both were trying to solicit sexual favors from him, and he was afraid that one or both had HIV/AIDS. See "Youth Guilty in the Killing of Two Gay Men," *New York Times,* February 11, 1995, p. A-7.

98. For instance, see Cleveland-Marshall College of Law, *AIDS: The Constitution and Public Health,* 24.

99. Don Bean and Katherine L. Siemon, "Jury Clears Hospital in AIDS Virus Privacy Suit," *Cleveland Plain Dealer,* May 5, 1990, p. 1-B.

100. See Arthur S. Leonard, "AIDS in the Workplace," in Harlon L. Dalton and Scott Burris, eds., *AIDS and the Law: A Guide for the Public* (New Haven, CT: Yale University Press, 1987).

101. One very unusual case involves a jury in West Virginia that awarded $2 million to a hospital guard because of negligence on the part of West Virginia University Hospitals. The guard was bitten by a patient with HIV/AIDS in the emergency room. The hospital administration argued that (1) there are no documented cases of someone contracting HIV/AIDS through saliva and (2) the guard had been tested for HIV on six occasions and was not yet seropositive. The guard claimed that, as a result of his being bitten by the patient, his wife divorced him and he was ostracized by the rest of his family. The jury found the hospital "95 percent negligible" for not informing the guard of the patient's condition. See *Johnson v. West Virginia University Hospitals,* No. 89-C-109 (W.Va.Cir.Ct. Monongalia County, December 13, 1989).

4. Attitudes toward HIV/AIDS in the Workplace

1. For instance, see Frederick C. Mosher, *Democracy and the Public Service* (New York: Oxford University Press, 1982); Donald S. Van Meter and Carl E. Van Horn, "The Policy Implementation Process: A Conceptual Framework," *Administration and Society* 6 (February 1975): 440–452.

2. For instance, see Harrell R. Rodgers, Jr., and Charles S. Bullock III, *Coercion to Compliance* (Lexington, MA: Lexington Books, 1976).

3. For instance, see Grace Hall Saltzstein, "Personnel Directors and Female Employment Representation: A New Addition to Models of Equal Employment Opportunity Policy?" *Social Science Quarterly* 64 (Spring 1983): 734–746; Frank J. Thompson, "Civil Servants and the Deprived: Sociopolitical and Occupational Explanations of Attitudes Toward Minority Hiring," *American Journal of Political Science* 22 (March 1978): 325–347; Frank J. Thompson and Bonnie Browne, "Commitment to the Disadvantaged Among Urban Administrators," *Urban Affairs Quarterly* 13 (March 1978): 355–377; Charles S. Bullock III and Charles M. Lamb, "Conditions Associated with Policy Implementation," in Charles S. Bullock III and Charles M. Lamb, eds., *Implementation of Civil Rights Policy* (Monterey, CA: Brookes/Cole, 1984): 184–208; and James D. Slack and Lee Sigelman, "City Managers and Affirmative Action: Testing a Model of Linkage," *Western Political Quarterly* 41 (December 1987): 673–684.

4. Frank J. Thompson, *Personnel Policy in the City* (Berkeley, CA: University of California Press, 1975), 7–8.

5. Response bias is the tendency to answer all questionnaire items in one category or value—by responding to all items with "agree," for instance, or with "strongly disagree." People who fill out a questionnaire in this way often do so as a result of fatigue.

6. International City and County Management Association, *Yearbook* (Washington, DC:

International City and County Management Association, 1994). The first mailing was sent to the city hall in 1,000 communities. Twelve questionnaires were returned because of nonexistent addresses, and seventeen were returned because the chief administrative officer did not want to participate in the survey.

7. Including a business card was done to increase the credibility of the study. See James D. Slack, "Maximizing Response Rates Among Local Public Officials: A Note About an Experiment with Business Cards," *Southeastern Political Review* (Spring 1989): 143–157.

8. The response rate is acceptable, given that (1) the topic is controversial, (2) questionnaires included an identification number, and (3) each copy of the questionnaire was sent to the person's business address. These factors tend to reduce the rates of response substantially. See Delbert C. Miller, *Handbook of Research Design and Social Measurement,* 5th ed. (Newbury Park, CA: Sage, 1991), 145–155.

9. Caucasians were 96.3 percent; men were 80.2 percent; and the average age was 47 years old. Eighty percent held college degrees: 35.7 percent bachelors, 20.6 percent the master in public administration (MPA), and 23.7 percent other graduate degrees (n = 490).

10. Very liberal = 1.0 percent; liberal = 15.5 percent; moderate = 51.2 percent; conservative = 30.0 percent; very conservative = 2.3 percent (n = 510).

11. Population ranges from 2,220 to 750,000.

12. Rural setting = 45.3 percent, suburban setting = 39.8 percent, urban setting = 14.9 percent (n = 517).

13. Because the two pieces of federal legislation offer identical protection, the survey used only the term "ADA." Attitudes about implementation of the ADA presumably extend to the Rehab Act as well.

5. Workplace Policies and Procedures

1. The typology is adapted from William J. Petak, "Emergency Management: A Challenge for Public Administration," *Public Administration Review* 45 (January 1985): 3–7 (special issue). Also see Roger E. Kasperson and K. David Pijawka, "Society Response to Hazards and Major Hazard Events: Comparing Natural and Technological Hazards," *Public Administration Review* 45 (January 1985): 7–18 (special issue).

2. For an excellent review, see Daniel C. McCool, *Public Policy Theories, Models, and Concepts: An Anthology* (Englewood Cliffs, NJ: Prentice-Hall, 1995). Also see Frank J. Thompson, "The Politics of Public Personnel Administration," and Alan Saltstein, "Personnel Management in the Local Government Setting," both in Steven W. Hays and Richard C. Kearney, eds., *Public Personnel Administration,* 3d ed. (Englewood Cliffs, NJ: Prentice-Hall, 1995).

3. Harrison M. Trice and Janice M. Beyer, *The Cultures of Work Organizations* (Englewood Cliffs, NJ: Prentice-Hall, 1993), 225.

4. For instance, see Jeffrey L. Pressman and Aaron B. Wildavsky, *Implementation* (Berkeley: University of California Press, 1973); Donald S. Van Meter and Carl E. Van Horn, "The Policy Implementation Process: A Conceptual Framework," *Administration and Society* 6 (February 1975): 246–275; and Jon Yinger, "States to the Rescue? Aid to Central Cities Under the New Federalism," *Public Budgeting and Finance* 10 (Summer 1990): 31–44.

5. On antidiscrimination policies, see Charles S. Bullock and Charles U. Lamb, *Implementation of Civil Rights Policy* (Monterey, CA: Brooks/Cole, 1984); on school desegregation, see Harrell R. Rodgers and Charles S. Bullock III, *Coercion to Compliance* (Lexington, MA: Lexington Books, 1976); on protected groups, see Grace H. Saltztein, "Female Mayors and Women in Municipal Jobs," *American Journal of Political Science* 30 (February 1986): 140–164.

6. See Frank J. Thompson, "Civil Servants and the Deprived: Sociopolitical and Occupational Explanations of Attitudes Toward Minority Hiring," *American Journal of Political Science*

22 (March 1978): 325–347; James D. Slack, "Affirmative Action and City Managers: Attitudes Toward Recruitment of Women," *Public Administration Review* 47 (March/April 1987): 199–206; N. Joseph Cayer and Roger L. Schaefer, "Affirmative Action and Municipal Employees," *Social Science Quarterly* 62 (September 1981): 487–494.

7. For instance, see James D. Slack, "Affirmative Action and City Managers"; and Peter K. Eisinger, "Black Employment in Municipal Jobs: The Impact of Black Political Power," *American Political Science Review* 76 (June 1982): 380–392.

8. For instance, see James D. Slack, "Information, Training, and Assistance Needs of Municipal Governments," *Public Administration Review* 50 (July/August 1990): 450–457.

9. See David R. Morgan, *Managing Urban America* (Pacific Grove, CA: Brooks/Cole, 1989).

10. For instance, see James D. Slack, "Local Government Training and Education Needs: Gearing Up for the Twenty-first Century," *Public Productivity and Management Review* 13 (Summer 1990): 397–404.

11. See Theodore H. Poister and Gregory Streib, "Management Tools in Municipal Government: Trends over the Past Decade," *Public Administration Review* 49 (May/June 1989): 240–248.

12. For instance, see Don A. Dillman and Kenneth R. Tremblay, Jr., "The Quality of Life in Rural America," *Annals of the American Academy of Political and Social Science* 49 (January 1977): 115–129.

13. For instance, see Leonard Cole, "Electing Blacks to Municipal Office: Structural and Social Determinants," *Urban Affairs Quarterly* 10 (September 1974): 17–39; and James D. Slack, "Affirmative Action and City Managers."

14. In the affirmative action literature, see Peter K. Eisinger, "Black Employment in Municipal Jobs"; Thomas Dye and J. Renick, "Political Power and City Jobs: Determinants of Minority Employment," *Social Science Quarterly* 58 (March 1977): 475–486; Grace Hall Saltzstein, "Personnel Directors and Female Employment Representation: A New Addition to Models of Equal Employment Opportunity Policy?" *Social Science Quarterly* 64 (1983): 734–746.

15. For instance, see Helen Gasch, Michael Poulson, Robert E. Fullilove, and Mindy Thompson Fullilove, "Shaping AIDS Education and Prevention Programs from African Americans Amidst Community Decline," *Journal of Negro Education* 60 (1991): 85–96.

16. For instance, see Herbert Kaufman, *Time, Chance, and Organizations: Natural Selection in a Perilous Environment* (Chatham, NJ: Chatham House, 1985); and Hal F. Rainey, "Public Management: Recent Research on the Political Context and Managerial Roles, Structures, and Behaviors," *Journal of Management* 15 (April): 229–250.

17. Nicholas Henry, *Public Administration and Public Affairs* (Englewood Cliffs, NJ: Prentice-Hall, 1995), 66.

18. For instance, see Jack P. DeSario, Sue R. Faerman, and James D. Slack, *Local Government Information and Training Needs in the Twenty-first Century* (Westport, CT: Quorum Books, 1994); and Cheryl Clark, "Is County Steering Some Away from AIDS Tests? Doctor Says 'Low Risk' Dissuaded to Save Funds," *San Diego Union Tribune,* October 10, 1992, p. B1.

19. See David R. Morgan, *Managing Urban America* (Pacific Grove, CA: Brooks/Cole, 1989); Irene S. Rubin, "Municipal Enterprises: Exploring Budgetary and Political Implications," *Public Administration Review* 48 (January/February 1988): 542–550; Glenn Abney and Thomas P. Lauth, *The Politics of State and City Administration* (Albany: State University of New York Press, 1986); and Theodore H. Poister and Gregory Streib, "Management Tools in Municipal Government."

20. For instance, see David R. Morgan, *Managing Urban America;* and Glenn Abney and Thomas P. Lauth, *The Politics of State and City Administration.*

21. Herbert A. Simon, *Administrative Behavior* (New York: Free Press, 1976).

22. For instance, see Frank Levy, Arnold Meltsner, and Aaron Wildavsky, *Urban Outcomes* (Berkeley: University of California Press, 1974); Bryan D. Jones, *Governing Urban America* (Boston: Little, Brown, 1983); J. Edward Kellough, *Equal Employment Opportunity Policy and Numeri-*

cal Goals and Timetables (New York: Praeger, 1989); and James D. Slack, "Women, Minorities, and Public Employer Attitudes: The Case of Fire Chiefs and Affirmative Action," *Public Administration Quarterly* 13 (Fall 1989): 388–411.

23. See William J. Petak, "Emergency Management: A Challenge for Public Administration," 1–172. Actually one needs only to compare the snow removal abilities of, say, the city of Dallas and the city of Minneapolis to see that greater experience with a crisis can promote improved management of the same kind of crisis in the future.

24. See Ronald O. Valdiserri and Gary R. West, "Barriers to the Assessment of Unmet Needs in Planning HIV/AIDS Prevention Programs," *Public Administration Review* 54 (January/February 1994): 25–30; and Richard J. Koehler, "HIV Infection, TB, and the Health Crisis in Corrections," *Public Administration Review* 54 (January/February 1994): 31–35.

25. All scales are "additive" scales; values are added across each item in the scale. Cronbach's alpha is used to determine the internal consistency of each scale.

26. These suggestions are specifically mentioned in the ADA, the *Congressional Record,* and the Equal Employment Opportunity Commission's *Interpretive Guidelines.* Transfers to other work areas are not mentioned in either the ADA or related documentation as a reasonable option for job applicants. They have therefore been omitted from the job applicant scale.

27. The following indicators are used for each factor. Personal characteristics: race, ideology, gender, age, education, belief that an HIV/AIDS plan is needed, supportive workplace attitudes, nonsupportive workplace attitudes, knowledge about the ADA, knowledge about HIV/AIDS. Organizational environment: rural/suburban/urban setting of the community, form of government, staff size, citizen opposition to hiring HIV/AIDS individuals, and council concern for hiring people with HIV/AIDS. Workplace experience: estimate of the number of workers with HIV/AIDS and experience in dealing with HIV/AIDS situations.

28. Multicollinearity is a state in which two indicators are actually measuring the same thing. In order to ensure that the independent variables are, indeed, "independent" of one another, variables should be selected that are not highly correlated. If they are highly correlated with each other, at least at the level of 0.7, then multicollinearity exists and one of the independent variables should be dropped from analysis. In this case, correlation between the two workplace attitude scales is 0.49.

29. The analysis used the SPSS-X procedure "Reliability." According to *SPSS-X User's Guide* (New York: McGraw-Hill, 1983), this procedure "performs an item analysis on the components of additive scales by computing commonly used coefficients of reliability" (p. 717).

30. For further discussion, see Edward G. Carmines and Richard A. Zellar, *Reliability and Validity Assessment,* Sage University Paper 17 (Beverly Hills, CA: Sage, 1981), 45.

31. In New Mexico, for instance, every municipality has established the position of ADA specialist.

32. I am assuming that 1 percent of the municipal workforce is in the HIV spectrum, the same proportion that might exist in the general public. If so, then there is an average of 2.08 seropositive workers, and not the estimated 0.71, on each city's workforce. The 2.08 calculation is 1 percent of the 208 average full-time municipal employees reported by practitioners responding to the questionnaire.

33. See Frederick C. Mosher, *Democracy and the Public Service.*

34. For instance, many changes in the curriculum standards for Master of Public Administration (MPA) programs have been instituted by the National Association of Schools of Public Affairs and Administration (NASPAA).

35. The four basic steps in the emergency management process are enumerated at the start of this chapter.

36. For the average 2.08 seropositive individuals estimated to work for each municipality, city hall needs to plan for the eventual expenditure of approximately $436,000 (with self-insurance) or

approximately $284,000 (with group health insurance). These expenditures are based on workplace costs as estimated in Chapter 2. Expenditures are assumed to be spread over a thirteen-year period. Costs are based on an annual salary of $25,000. Estimated cost, especially for sick-day utilization, varies by salary.

6. HIV/AIDS and the Public Service: The Crisis Revisited

1. LRP Publications, which publishes the journal *AIDS Policy and Law,* offers a sixty-six-page pamphlet on recent court rulings about HIV in the workplace. The pamphlet is titled "AIDS in the Workplace: Evolving Issues and Court Cases" and can be ordered by calling 800-341-7874, ext. 274. See also Laura Duncan, "Illinois Ranks Fourth in ADA Complaints, EEOC Says," *Chicago Daily Law Bulletin,* October 27, 1994, p. 1.

2. Approximately 47,000 Americans died in the Vietnam War.

3. Approximately 292,000 Americans died as a result of World War II. Consequently there were approximately 292,000 American homes that affixed gold stars in their windows to signify a World War II–related death in the family. If we did the same today for all the sons and daughters who have been (or are destined to be) lost as a result of contracting full-blown AIDS, then there would be over half a million homes with gold stars in the windows.

4. Approximately 365,000 Americans died in that war.

5. For instance, see the November 10, 1994, press release of the Gay Men's Health Crisis on the appointment of Patsy Fleming as National AIDS Coordinator.

6. The staff provides referral assistance to other agencies, such as the EEOC or the CDC.

7. For instance, the staff at the National AIDS Hotline is not aware of *any* federal agencies that provide workplace assistance.

8. For instance, see William J. Petak, "Emergency Management: A Challenge for Public Administration," *Public Administration Review* 45 (January 1985): 3–6 (special issue); Louise K. Comfort, "Integrating Organizational Action in Emergency Management: Strategies for Change," *Public Administration Review* 45 (January 1985): 155–164; David McLoughlin, "A Framework for Integrated Emergency Management," *Public Administration Review* 45 (January 1985): 165–172; Roger E. Kasperson and K. David Pijawka, "Society Response to Hazards and Major Hazard Events: Comparing Natural and Technological Hazards," *Public Administration Review* 45 (January 1985): 7–18.

9. Since the first edition of this book, the U.S. Centers for Disease Control and Prevention has also developed a model plan. See Appendix C.

10. See James D. Slack, "Managing the Workplace Ramifications of Human Immunodeficiency Virus (HIV) and Acquired Immunodeficiency Syndrome (AIDS) for Public Agencies and Health Care Facilities in the Southern San Joaquin Valley, California" (Public Service Institute, California State University, Bakersfield, summer 1995); and James D. Slack and Anelia Luna, "A Model Plan for Managing the Workplace Ramifications of Acquired Immunodeficiency Syndrome (AIDS) for Municipalities in Cuyahoga County and Northwestern Ohio" (Center for Governmental Research and Public Service, Bowling Green State University, Bowling Green, Ohio, November 1992).

11. Most workplaces, including municipalities, do not take advantage of the best source of information on HIV/AIDS, the Gay Men's Health Crisis (GMHC). This is the oldest and most experienced counseling center in the U.S. The GMHC can answer questions about many aspects of the HIV/AIDS crisis, from modes of transmission and safer-sex practices to the legalities of HIV antibody blood testing in the workplace. It can also provide information about community-based HIV/AIDS organizations in every metropolitan area. (The GMHC can be reached at 212-807-6655.)

12. For instance, see the *American Red Cross Workplace HIV/AIDS Instructor's Manual*

(Washington, DC: American Red Cross, 1992); and Alan Emery, *How to Implement a Workplace HIV/AIDS Education Program: Employee HIV/AIDS Education* (Washington, DC: American Red Cross and the U.S. Centers for Disease Control, 1992).

13. See chapter 3, "Training Theory and Approaches," in Jack P. DeSario, Sue R. Faerman, and James D. Slack, *Local Government Information and Training Needs in the Twenty-first Century* (Westport, CT: Quorum Books, 1994), 37–54.

14. For instance, see "Readers' Forum on AIDS in Workplace," *PA Times* 15 (February 1, 1992): 9.

15. William J. Petak, "Emergency Management," 4.

16. William J. Petak, "Emergency Management," 4.

Index

Acquired Immunodeficiency Syndrome (AIDS): czar, 98, 115; demographic trends, 11, 12; estimates of infection in the United States, 11; "full blown," 5; phobia, 70

Acute HIV, 5

AIDS Coalition to Unleash Power (ACT-UP), 30

Americans with Disabilities Act (ADA): application to stages of HIV, 40; confidentiality, 50–51; definition of disability, 38–39; differences with Rehabilitation Act, 36–38; documentation requirements, 41; essential functions of the job, 41, 42; management's responsibilities, 41–53; notification requirements, 41; overview 21, 25; reasonable accommodations, 45–47; responsibilities of job applicant/employee with HIV/AIDS, 40–41; screening, 42–45; similarities with Rehabilitation Act, 38; substantially limiting impairments, 40; undue hardship, 47–49

Antiviral drugs, 6, 144 (n. 17)

Asymptomatic stage of HIV, 5

Attitudes of practitioners: applying the law in the workplace, 60–64; changes over time, 66–69; confidentiality, 65, 67; HIV testing, 64–66; understanding the law and HIV/AIDS, 58–60

Bureaucracy, external side: 15, 27–30, 93; delivery of services, 28; level/quality of services, 28, 29; manner of service delivery, 29, 30

Bureaucracy, internal side: contact between seropositive employees and citizens and coworkers, 34; estimate of government workforce with HIV, 28; government preparedness, 31; overview, 31, 93; practitioners' estimate of number of employees with HIV, 78–79; selection and screening of seropositive employees, 33. *See also* Preparedness

CD$_4$ T-cell, 2, 4, 5, 8, 10

Centers for Disease Control and Prevention (CDC), 5, 98

Civil/individual rights, 16–18

Conceptual framework for analysis of workplace preparedness, 71–74, 75

Confidentiality, 33–34; attitudes of practitioners, 65, 67; of HIV test results, 50–51

Court cases, major HIV/AIDS related: *Alexander v. Choate,* 48; *Chalk v. U.S. District Court, Central District of California,* 39; *Clarence B. Cain v. Joel Hyatt,* 49–50; *Doe v. Borough of Barrington,* 50; *Doe v. Charlotte Memorial Hospital,* 39; *Leckelt v. Board of Commission of Hospital District No. 1,* 39; *Little v. Bryce,* 50; *Saxton v. Vanzant,* 50; *School Board of Nassau County, Fla. v. Arline,* 39; *Thomas v. Atascadero Unified School District,* 39; *Thornburgh v. American College of Obstetricians and Gynecologists,* 50; *Whalen v. Roe,* 50

Deoxyribonucleic acids (DNA), 4, 5

Disability, defined, 38

Drug therapies, 6, 22

Emergency Management: HIV as a public emergency, 31–32; steps/procedures, 71, 100, 113

Employee Retirement Income Security Act (ERISA), 25

Equal Employment Opportunity Commission (EEOC), 25; definition of reasonable accommodation, 45–46; *Interpretive Guidelines* for undue hardship, 48–49

Federal government: coordinative policy, 114; distributive policy, 114; National AIDS Policy Office, 98–99, 114–15; regulative policy, 114; role in assisting workplaces, 111, 113–14

First amendment rights, 2

Gay-related immunodeficiency (GRID), 6

About the Author

James D. Slack is a professor of public administration and chair of the Department of Public Policy and Administration, School of Business and Public Administration, California State University at Bakersfield. He received his Ph.D. from Miami University in 1981. Professor Slack has been a policy and management consultant for numerous public and private organizations on issues relating to HIV/AIDS, antidiscrimination, and human resource needs and planning. In 1990 he was a member of the American delegation to the first Sino-American Symposium on the Management of HIV/AIDS in Beijing, China. He is author of over 30 articles, numerous book chapters, and books, including studies on the training and professional development needs of local governments and the workplace ramifications of HIV/AIDS. He won the Laverne Burchfield Award for his article "The Public Administration of AIDS" in 1993. Professor Slack lives in Bakersfield, California, with his wife, Janis, and their children, Sarah and Samuel.